Navicular Syndrome Explained

Also by David W. Ramey, DVM

The Anatomy of a Horse
Concise Guide to Arthritis in the Horse
Concise Guide to Colic in the Horse
Concise Guide to Laminitis in the Horse
Concise Guide to Medications and Supplements for the Horse
Concise Guide to Nutrition in the Horse
Concise Guide to Tendon and Ligament Injuries in the Horse
A Consumer's Guide to Alternative Therapies in the Horse
Horsefeathers: Fact vs. Myths about Your Horse's Health

HORSE HEALTH EXPLAINED

Navicular Syndrome Explained

David W. Ramey DVM

KENILWORTH PRESS

First published in 1997, under the title *Concise Guide to Navicular Syndrome in the Horse*, by Howell Book House, a Simon & Schuster Macmillan Company, New York, USA

This revised paperback edition published in 2002 by
Kenilworth Press Ltd
Addington
Buckingham
MK18 2JR

Published simultaneously in the USA, under the title *Concise Guide to Navicular Syndrome in the Horse*, by
Trafalgar Square Publishing
North Pomfret
Vermont 05053
USA

Disclaimer
This book is not to be used in place of veterinary care and expertise. The author and publisher shall have neither liability nor responsibility to any person or entity with respect to any loss or damage caused or alleged to be caused directly or indirectly by the information contained in this book. While the book is as accurate as the author can make it, there may be errors, omissions, and inaccuracies.

British Library Cataloguing in Publication Data
A CIP record for this book is available from the British Library

ISBN 1-872119-47-6

Printed and bound in Great Britain by Bell & Bain, Glasgow

CONTENTS

ACKNOWLEDGEMENTS

I am most grateful to Martha Cook and Caroline Robbins of Trafalgar Square Publishing, for their long-expressed interest and support. The fine ladies who reviewed the first edition of this book, Denise Leeper and Linda Rarey, were responsible for helping make the original content understandable—hopefully, the new additions, made with the gracious and invaluable help of Dr Kees Dik of the University of Utrecht, Dr Bill Moyer of Texas A&M University and Dr Steve O'Grady of Northern Virginia Equine, will be equally useful and easy to comprehend. Lynda Fennemann's illustrations needed no revision – they were perfect the first time. To Madelyn Larsen, who first gave me my start – thanks for all of the advice and encouragement. Finally, to Jackson and Aidan, thanks for making me smile every day.

INTRODUCTION

Navicular syndrome: it is likely that no condition of the horse's limbs is mentioned as frequently by horse owners as is navicular syndrome. No other condition seems to be as frequently suspected as a cause of lameness in the horse as disease of the navicular bone. Certainly, few conditions that cause lameness in the horse are as frequently diagnosed by veterinary surgeons, farriers, and amateur-observers-with-too-much-time-on-their-hands as is navicular syndrome. Navicular disease is a headache for everyone.

However, in the author's opinion, much of this fuss is unwarranted. That's because, while navicular syndrome is certainly a serious condition that can cause lameness in the horse, it is also a condition that is frequently over-diagnosed. It is the 'first diagnosis of the diagnostically destitute', according to one authority. Navicular syndrome in the horse is a serious condition. It requires a careful and thoughtful approach to diagnosis because the prognosis is not good. Treatment of this condition can be frustrating. However—and this is important—it is not the first condition that should be immediately considered when any horse shows signs of lameness. There's a good chance that the horse doesn't have it.

This book was written to try to help clear up many of the concerns and misconceptions about navicular syndrome in the horse. It will help show you what the condition is, and explain some of the current thoughts as to how the condition develops. The book will discuss the diagnosis and the many proposed treatments for the condition (many of which clearly don't work). It will show you why the diagnosis of disease of the navicular bone should not normally be an easy diagnosis to make. Hopefully, it will also help you understand why it is a diagnosis that is often easily made, even if that diagnosis isn't warranted.

With the information that you will gain from this book, you should be able to help participate in detecting the cause of your horse's lameness. Should your horse be diagnosed as having navicular syndrome, with the help of the book you should be able to help select and understand a treatment. Finally, based on what you learn here, you should be able to make some realistic decisions about your horse's future.

Navicular syndrome is not what you probably think. Like any problem, it is one that needs to be approached rationally. If your horse has been diagnosed with navicular syndrome, don't panic. With the help of this book, you can approach your horse's lameness with thoughtfulness and understanding, and you'll figure out what to do.

1

Some Normal Anatomy and Physiology of the Horse's Foot as it Relates to Navicular Syndrome

Frankly, anatomy can be pretty boring stuff. And, to the dismay of freshmen veterinary students everywhere, you get a solid year of it in veterinary school. However, before you can begin to understand what navicular syndrome in the horse is (and is not), you have to understand what and where the navicular bone is found. Familiarizing yourself with the anatomy of the horse's foot is essential to understanding the problem of navicular syndrome. What follows is not a complete anatomic description of the foot; that would be too time-consuming, technical and tedious for this book. You don't need to know everything anyway. Instead, most of the important anatomical features of this area that pertain to the navicular bone are highlighted. There is enough basic anatomy and physiology information here so that you can ultimately begin to figure out the basis for this problematic condition of the horse's foot (and hopefully not so much as to make you crazy).

THE BONES, TENDONS AND LIGAMENTS OF THE HORSE'S HOOF

The Bones of the Foot

Bone is the framework upon which the horse's body is built. Happily, there are only three bones that make up the framework of the horse's foot.

The only bone that is really obvious to the naked eye on a standing horse is the so-called short pastern bone (called the second phalanx by anatomists). You can see it because even though it helps make up the framework of the foot, most of the short pastern bone is not contained inside the hoof. However, the bottom (ground) surface of this bone makes up the top part of the joint of the foot. The bone itself also serves as the attachment for some very important ligaments.

Below the short pastern bone (towards the ground) and contained within the hoof itself is the second of the three important bones of the horse's foot: the third or distal phalanx. This bone is known to horse people as the 'coffin' bone because, as was noted in the 1700s, it is contained in the hoof like a buried coffin. The coffin bone meshes with the short pastern bone that sits above it and helps form the joint of the foot.

The coffin bone has a rather unique shape. As you might suspect, the leading edge of the bone is shaped in an arc, just like the horse's hoof. But if you cut through the hoof parallel to the ground and look down from the top, you'll see that the entire coffin bone is shaped like a quarter moon, with the outside curve of the moon being the leading edge of the foot.

Lying just above and within the inside curve of the quarter moon you'll find the distal sesamoid bone, commonly known as the navicular bone (the source of your concern). The word 'navicular' comes from the Latin word for boat. Perhaps, when you look at the bone on an X-ray, you can imagine the keel of a boat. (See Figures 4a and 4b, p. 42.) It's rather amazing that such a little bone can cause such big problems, isn't it?

The Joint of the Foot

Any point in the horse's body where two bones meet is called a joint. The ends of the bones that meet in joints are covered with a unique substance called cartilage. Cartilage provides a smooth, almost frictionless gliding surface for the bones to slide against each other. It also helps cushion the ends of the bones when the weight of the horse squeezes them together. Inside the joint, a fluid (the synovial fluid) is produced that provides nutrition to the cartilage cells and helps lubricate the joint. The lining cells of the joint capsule, which surrounds the joint, produce this fluid. The joint capsule is the wrapping paper that surrounds the package that is the whole joint.

The joint of the foot (the 'coffin' joint) is made up of the contacting surfaces of all three of the bones of the foot that you have just learned about (see Figure 1). The surfaces of all these bones are intimately associated with each other. Of course, the fluid in the coffin joint is in contact with the surface of all three of the bones at some point.

This close contact helps explain why it can sometimes be extremely difficult (even impossible) for someone (like your veterinary surgeon) to precisely distinguish between the various bones and joint surfaces when there is a problem in the horse's heel or foot area. They're all extremely close together—it's not like trying to figure out whether the problem is in the nose or the tail. The joint fluid that touches one bone touches them all. This close proximity has some important implications for the diagnosis of problems in this area, as

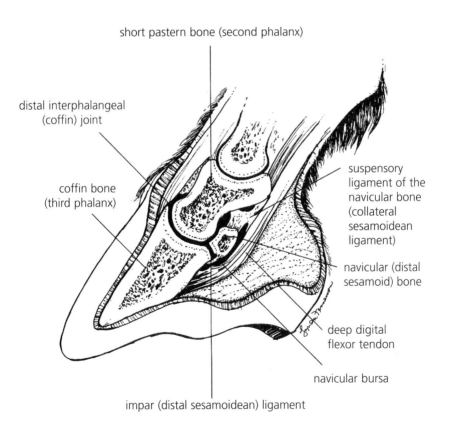

Figure 1. Cross-section of foot as seen from the side.

you will see in later chapters.

Of particular importance to people who are interested in navicular syndrome (of which you, presumably, are one) is the structure of the joint of the foot in the area of the navicular bone. The navicular bone is not normally a smooth structure. It has little pits, depressions and surface irregularities in it. These irregularities occur where the navicular bone makes contact with the lining of the coffin joint. The coffin joint lining can even make little indentations into the navicular bone. These fossae (as the depressions are called) can frequently be seen on X-rays. There is a great deal of discussion in the veterinary community about the significance of these fossae in relation to navicular syndrome. Many of them can occur in navicular bones that are simply normal (much more on them later).

The Ligaments of the Foot

Ligaments are supporting structures that, in the case of the foot (as well as in most other areas), connect bone to bone. Ligaments are stabilizing straps of connective tissue. Their function is to try to keep the bones in a constant relationship to each other. (If you placed two boxes next to each other and taped the sides so that the boxes would stay together, the tape would be serving the same function for the boxes as ligaments do for bone.) For example, there are collateral ligaments of the foot that run along both sides of the coffin and short pastern bones. Of much more interest (at least in regard to how ligaments pertain to navicular syndrome) are two other ligaments that attach to the navicular bone (see Figure 2).

The suspensory ligaments of the navicular bone (called the collateral sesamoidean ligaments by anatomists) start out from little depressions on either side of the long pastern bone (also known as the first phalanx). The long pastern bone is located immediately above the short pastern bone (second phalanx). One ligament curves around and behind each side of the short pastern bone and attaches to each end, as well as to the top side, of the navicular bone. Branches of these ligaments also attach to the coffin bone. These ligaments effectively suspend the navicular bone in its spot (hence the name 'suspensory'), which, as you know, is tucked in behind the coffin bone and just below the short pastern bone.

The bottom of the navicular bone is attached to the bottom of the coffin bone by the impar ligament (the distal sesamoidean ligament). The impar ligament is a short structure that begins at the bottom (distal) border of the navicular bone and ties into the coffin bone on its ground side, just under where the large deep flexor tendon joins into the coffin bone.

The Deep Flexor Tendon

Tendons connect muscles to bone. When a muscle contracts (contracting is the only thing a muscle can do), it causes the bone to move via the tendon. The tendon transmits the force of the contracting muscle to the bone. (Of course, tendons have many other

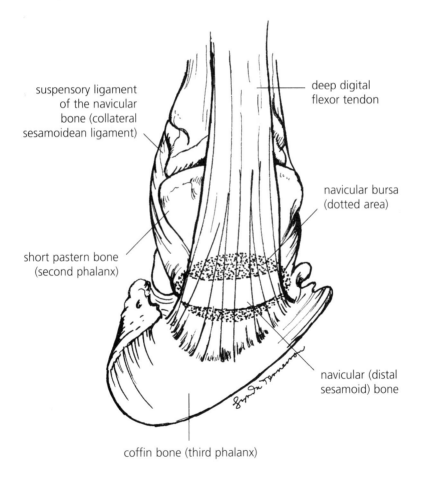

suspensory ligament of the navicular bone (collateral sesamoidean ligament)

deep digital flexor tendon

navicular bursa (dotted area)

short pastern bone (second phalanx)

navicular (distal sesamoid) bone

coffin bone (third phalanx)

Figure 2. View of foot from below and off to the side, with the hoof removed.

important functions. That is the sort of stuff found in *The Concise Guide to Tendon and Ligament Injuries in the Horse* (published by John Wiley & Son, USA). Of concern in the whole muddy picture that is navicular syndrome is a large, important tendon that runs down the back of the horse's leg. This is the tendon of the deep digital flexor muscle, commonly called the deep digital flexor tendon.

The deep flexor tendon begins at the level of the horse's knee (carpus) and descends down the back of the lower limb (or digit; hence the term 'digital'). It can easily be felt down in the area behind the horse's cannon bone as well as lower, behind the pastern. It continues on down underneath the heel of the foot and travels directly under the bottom of the navicular bone. The tendon then inserts into the coffin bone (and right over the top of the impar ligament of the navicular bone).

The Navicular Bursa
Sitting between the deep digital flexor tendon and the navicular bone is the navicular bursa. A bursa is a fluid-filled sac. Bursas are found in various locations in the horse's body, in fact, they occur just about anywhere a tendon makes a turn over the top of a bone. For example, there's an important bursa in your shoulder where the tendons make the turn to run down your arm. A bursa is like a little pillow that helps to cushion a tendon where it makes a turn. The navicular bursa in the horse helps to cushion the deep flexor tendon as it makes its turn over the top of the navicular bone.

Some vets think that the navicular bursa is the source of many of the problems that are involved with navicular syndrome. Its actual role in navicular syndrome is a subject for discussion and is still under investigation. (There's more on this subject later.)

The Nerve Supply to the Navicular Bone
The nerves that give feeling to the navicular area are of great interest to those who study navicular syndrome. It's very important to understand the nerve supply to this crowded area of the horse's foot. There are two main reasons for this (besides just plain curiosity).

The first reason is for diagnostic purposes. As you will learn, one of the common diagnostic techniques used for determining whether or not a horse has navicular syndrome (or indeed, any type of lameness) is the nerve 'block'. Nerve blocks allow veterinary surgeons to try to determine the area that hurts by a process of elimination. To perform a nerve block, a veterinary surgeon may put a small amount of local anaesthetic over the nerves that go to an area; 'blocking' a nerve means that the horse won't have any feeling in the area that's supplied by that nerve. Alternatively, anaesthetic may be injected directly into a joint to numb it, and, in the case of the foot, a whole lot more. If the horse is limping because a particular area hurts and the area that hurts is made numb, hey presto, the horse will stop limping. You can then assume that the pain that caused the limp came from the numb area.

The problem is, in the foot, there's a whole lot of stuff in the small area that gets made numb when you shoot some anaesthetic over the top of the nerves. Obviously, to do the best job that you can at interpreting a nerve blocking procedure, it helps to know precisely where the nerves that you are 'blocking' go. Conversely, if you're not sure where the nerves go, you can't make a very accurate determination as to what the problem is. For example, if you made an entire lame leg numb and the horse then went sound, you might know that the leg hurt somewhere but you still wouldn't have any idea where. That's not particularly useful information. Similarly, on a smaller scale, this is the same problem that veterinary surgeons have to deal with in order to make an accurate diagnosis of navicular syndrome.

The second reason for knowing about the nerves of the navicular area is surgical. In horses that do not respond to any treatment for navicular syndrome, occasionally a surgical neurectomy (cutting the nerves) is recommended. Obviously, you have to know where the nerves are to find them, cut them, and understand what effect this is going to have on the horse.

There are two major nerves that travel down to the navicular bone (see Figure 3). These paired nerves are called the palmar digital nerves ('palmar' refers to the posterior aspect of the horse's front leg). They're most easily found running down the back of the horse's pastern. The nerves lie just to the side of the large deep digital flexor tendon and in close association with the major veins and arteries of the back of the foot. Importantly, these large nerves do not only supply the navicular bone; they also provide sensation to almost the entire foot of the horse. By blocking the sensation in these nerves with local anaesthetic, you remove the feeling to most of foot, not just to the navicular bone. This has important implications for the diagnosis of navicular syndrome.

At the level of the navicular bone itself, the nerve supply becomes quite complex. Most of the nerves that directly supply the navicular bone travel through the impar ligament below and the suspensory ligaments above. Here's where it gets complicated. The inner surface of these ligaments also makes up part of the lining for the joint of the foot (the coffin joint). This has important significance for the interpretation of local anaesthetic blocks of the coffin joint, as you will see in Chapter 4.

The nerve supply to the navicular bursa goes along a slightly different path. The nerves to the navicular bursa also travel through the impar and collateral sesamoidean ligaments, but on the opposite side (the ground side) from the nerves that go to the navicular bone itself.

paired palmar digital nerves

deep digital
flexor tendon

Figure 3. From behind the pastern, with the skin and superficial tissues removed, the palmar digital nerves can be seen. Note the deep flexor tendon running down the centre of the pastern.

Although the nerves that travel through this area mostly supply the navicular bursa, they also provide sensation to a small part of the surface of the deep flexor tendon where it runs over the bursa. It's also possible to put anaesthetic into the navicular bursa as part of a diagnostic work-up for navicular syndrome.

HOW THE FOOT MOVES

The coffin joint is what anatomists call a 'hinge' joint (actually, the term is ginglymus joint, but that's not exactly a conversational term and if you use the term, most people won't understand what you're trying to say and they'll think that you're talking down to them). It's called a hinge joint because when the joint moves, it opens and closes like the hinge on a door. It's the same type of movement that you have in your elbow, although in the joint of the horse's foot, obviously, there's a lot less movement.

The coffin joint is pulled up and forward (extended) by a large extensor tendon that attaches to the top and front of the coffin bone. It is pulled up and bent back (flexed) by the action of the tendon of the deep digital flexor muscle. The flexion action is most likely made easier by the location of the navicular bone. The deep digital flexor tendon makes a tight turn around the navicular bone (a turn that, as you remember, is cushioned by the navicular bursa). This turn in the tendon apparently allows the navicular bone to act like the fulcrum in a lever system. (If you use a bar to prise a rock up out of the ground, your work is made a lot easier if you put a piece of wood under the end of the bar to prise up against. That piece of wood is called the fulcrum.) The navicular bone may also act as a sort of pulley for the system. Finally, the location of the navicular bone may help ensure that, regardless of the orientation of the joint of the foot, the deep flexor tendon will always be inserted into the coffin bone at a constant angle, which is most efficient for movement of the limb. But whatever the true underlying function, there is no question that the navicular bone is an important stress point for the horse's entire foot.

When the horse's foot strikes the ground, in the majority of normal horses that have been studied, the heels (the back part of the foot) strike the ground first. (In the remainder of the horses studied, the foot lands flat.) The rest of the foot follows the heels onto the

17

ground in sequence, from the back of the foot to the front. The weight of the horse causes the hoof to be compressed and to spread out as it is mashed into the ground.

As the foot continues to bear weight, the structures of the foot are pushed downward into the ground. The force from the horse's weight passes directly through the navicular bone, the navicular bursa, the flexor tendon and the digital cushion of the foot. (The digital cushion is like a pillow that sits between all the sensitive structures inside the foot and the hard tissue that contacts the ground.) To accommodate the pressure, the foot expands. The expansion of the foot directs the forces to the outside edges of the foot. The forces then travel up and out of the hoof wall. (It's also interesting that additional shock absorption is actually provided by the blood in the horse's foot. The blood in the foot provides a cushion in the same manner that a waterbed does. Following the principle of hydraulics, the blood in the foot also helps to get rid of the stress that is applied to the foot by the horse's weight.)

When the full weight of the horse is on the foot and the structures of the foot have sunk as low as they can, the deep flexor muscle starts to act. It pulls on the bottom of the coffin bone (and over the top of the navicular bone). This causes an initial downward pull on the horse's toe. The whole foot begins to rotate down and starts getting pulled back and up. The navicular bone takes a tremendous amount of stress at this point—it's right in the centre of that rotation. As the horse continues to travel forward, his leg rolls over the toe of the foot and the entire foot structure comes up off the ground. The foot then travels through the air as the horse strides forward. Finally, the foot will hit the ground and begin the whole cycle all over again.

As you can imagine, the back part of the horse's foot (the heel) comes under a lot of stress in the course of a normal stride. Indeed, the horse's heel is a very sensitive area. There are a lot of reasons for this sensitivity. The heels are the shortest part of the foot and are found the closest to the ground. Because they are shorter, they are also softer than any other part of the foot (they haven't grown out enough to get as hard and dry as the rest of the foot). The heels also normally hit the ground first. Finally, research shows that they take a greater part of the force at impact on the ground than any other part of the foot. It's no wonder (and it's a fact) that this short, soft, stressed area of the horse's foot is the area that is most commonly affected by lameness!

Because the heels are so frequently involved as a cause of lameness in the horse and because there are so many structures that lie in the heel area, it's extremely important for you to remember one thing: *Not all lameness that originates in the horse's heels is associated with the navicular bone!* Injury to any one of the structures in the heels, including the digital cushion, the impar ligament, the suspensory ligaments of the navicular bone, the navicular bursa, the coffin joint, the coffin bone, or the navicular bone itself (among others) can be associated with lameness. Depending on your definition, any of these structures may be associated with navicular syndrome, too. (For the author's definition, read on.)

Navicular Syndrome Defined

When you try to come up with a concise definition for navicular syndrome, straight away you get into trouble. Believe it or not, there is no generally accepted definition of the term 'navicular syndrome' in the veterinary community. More than anything else, this reflects the fact that navicular syndrome is a complex and poorly understood condition. If it were easy to understand, it would be easy to define (and easy to recognize and probably easier to treat).

As a matter of fact, there's not even general agreement about calling the condition navicular syndrome. Many people refer to the problems that occur in and around the horse's navicular bone as navicular disease.

What's the difference? Well, in some ways it's a matter of semantics. But if you look deeper, it's apparent that this is not a mere semantic issue. Disease is, by definition, 'a definite morbid process having a characteristic train of symptoms' (*Dorland's Illustrated Medical Dictionary*, 25th Edition, W. B. Saunders Co., Philadelphia, 1974). Thus, to call problems associated in and around the horse's navicular bone a 'disease' is to imply that the condition has a regular and recognizable set of factors that occur with it. When you think of a 'disease', you think of a well-wrapped package of clinical signs, diagnostic elements and treatments.

With abnormalities in and around the navicular bone, however, you have anything but a neat package of events. Therefore, in the minds of many veterinarians (the author included), the use of the term 'disease' to describe what's going on in and around the horse's navicular bone isn't appropriate. A better term to describe the condition is 'syndrome'.

A syndrome is, by definition, 'a set of symptoms which occur together' (*Dorland's*). It's a much more general term than 'disease'.

By calling the problems that occur in and around the horse's navicular bone a 'syndrome', veterinary surgeons acknowledge that they don't know exactly what's going on. The use of the word 'syndrome' implies that you are dealing with a complex condition, one that many have many potential treatments.

Of course, once you've decided to call it something, then you have to decide what that something is. With navicular syndrome, that's the hard part. Navicular syndrome may actually involve a complex of diseases and injuries that affect the heel area of the horse's foot. The reasons that these diseases and injuries occur are poorly understood. There may be many factors involved. In its broadest terms, navicular syndrome may involve a number of structures, including (among other structures) the navicular bone, the navicular bursa, the blood supply to the area, the joint of the foot (the coffin joint), the ligaments of the navicular bone, and the deep digital flexor tendon.

However, some veterinary surgeons prefer a more narrow definition for the term navicular syndrome. They feel that the term specifically refers to a condition that only involves the horse's navicular bone and one of the other associated structures. For example, these vets feel that a navicular ligament problem is completely different from a problem involving the navicular bone. They think the two conditions should be considered separately. And, in many ways, they're right. The prognosis for recovery from a ligament injury is most likely completely different from that of a problem involving degeneration of the navicular bone itself. The challenge for veterinary medicine (and veterinary surgeons), then, is in trying to distinguish between the various things that can cause soreness in the heel area of the horse, the area where the navicular bone lies. So far, that's not something veterinary medicine can do very well.

What does the author of this book think? The philosophy of this book is that a more narrow definition of the term navicular syndrome is appropriate. That is, the use of the term navicular syndrome should be confined to those horses in which disease of the navicular bone itself can be reasonably suggested. Otherwise, even broader terms, such as heel soreness or caudal (refers to the back part of the foot) foot soreness, or even 'foot pain' can be used to describe horses that have poorly defined lameness originating from the back part of the foot.

To the author, the term 'navicular syndrome' implies a chronic, incurable condition associated with deterioration of the navicular bone. In his practice, and when appropriate, by using the term 'heel soreness' or 'caudal foot pain' instead of 'navicular syndrome', the author attempts to distinguish between the horses that have an incurable condition (long-term deterioration of the navicular bone) and those horses that may be able to recover from their problems. In fact, given the large number of structures involved in and the complex anatomy of the horse's heel, the odds are that a particular horse with pain in the back part of the foot does not have pain specifically coming from the navicular bone. In the author's mind, calling all horses with heel pain of undetermined cause 'navicular' is painting them all with a very broad and damning brush. In the author's experience, most horses with deep heel pain of undetermined cause get better; most horses with navicular syndrome do not.

Don't despair if you find all of this a bit confusing. Unfortunately, it almost has to be. At this point in time, it's confusing to everyone. The development, diagnosis and treatment of navicular syndrome isn't well understood by anyone. There isn't even a consensus in the veterinary community about what the syndrome is. Navicular syndrome is not a nice, neat package. Therefore, it is predictable that you will hear all sorts of opinions about navicular syndrome in the horse. Conflicting, sometimes almost opposing, statements can be heard from individuals who are well educated and well respected in the veterinary field. At this time, there is no single right solution to the problem of navicular syndrome.

Thus, in a way, even the title of this book is a bit of an oxymoron. There is no concise box into which navicular syndrome can fit. However, it is possible to understand what navicular syndrome is and what it is not. It is possible to make some rational treatment decisions for your horse. You can make reasonable predictions about what is going to happen to horses that are truly affected with the navicular syndrome, as well as for horses that have pain coming from other structures. The following chapters should help you do just that.

Navicular Syndrome: Pathology and Theories of Development

A number of theories have been developed in an effort to understand the underlying cause of navicular syndrome. They're not really all that technical and they're interesting, even if they are unproven. After all, it is somewhat important for veterinary surgeons to try to work out why the problem occurs. If you could get to the root cause of navicular syndrome, then you could make some reasonable recommendations for prevention or treatment.

Unfortunately (at least for those of you who like easy answers), when it comes to navicular syndrome, the word 'multifactorial' comes to mind. That means there may not be a single cause of the problem. That also means, of course, that there may be no single solution, either. Some part of each of the many theories of development of navicular syndrome may contribute to the condition itself.

ISCHAEMIC THEORY

Ischaemia is defined as a loss or lack of blood supply to an area. In 1979, it was proposed that navicular syndrome in the horse was caused by problems in the circulation of blood to the navicular bone. This theory proposed that, in horses with navicular syndrome, little blood clots formed in the small arteries running to the navicular bone. These clots would block the normal circulation of blood to the bone. As a result, there would be pain resulting from the loss of circulation and bone death in the area supplied by the little arteries that were plugged up by the clots. (It would resemble what happens in the process of heart disease in people.)

If, as a result of the proposed ischaemia, bone began to die (which would be the normal response to the loss of circulation), the horse's body would have to remove the dying bone. This could then leave a navicular bone with little holes in it from where dead bone was removed. That might explain the typical X-ray changes that are seen in the bones of horses with navicular syndrome (more on that later).

Unfortunately, at least insofar as support for this theory goes, nobody has been able to show that this theoretical situation is what actually happens. When navicular bones from horses that have had navicular syndrome are looked at under the microscope, nobody has been able to find any blood clots in the little arteries, or areas of bone dying from lack of circulation.

If this ischaemic theory were true, at least some part of effective treatment would logically be aimed at affecting the horse's circulation. However, as you will see, even though the ischaemic theory of navicular syndrome can't be supported based on the scientific evidence, some component of navicular syndrome may ultimately involve the circulation of blood in or to the bone. In fact, some treatment to affect the circulation to the horse's foot is a commonly travelled avenue of therapy for navicular syndrome.

MECHANICAL THEORIES

Mechanical theories for the development of navicular syndrome suggest that the condition develops due to physical stress on the horse's foot, particularly in the heel area. That is, due to some combination of poorly defined factors, there are abnormal stresses applied to the horse's foot. For example, things such as too much galloping on hard ground or abnormal forces applied to a young horse's limbs due to neglected and unbalanced feet, might cause such stresses. Whatever the underlying cause, these mechanical stresses may ultimately result in changes to the navicular bone. Interestingly, from a therapeutic standpoint, the mechanical theories suggest that if you can improve the way that the horse's foot moves, you may be able to help relieve the stress on the foot and thereby treat the condition.

Most people don't realize that bone is active, living tissue. Like most other tissues in the horse's body, it is constantly replacing itself as cells wear out. Because it is living and continually changing, bone also responds to stress. When pressure (stress) is applied to bone, the bone responds by increasing its activity; this is called remodelling. Stress causes old bone to be removed and causes new bone to be added at a more rapid pace than would normally occur. Stressed areas of bone generally also become thicker over time. And, interestingly, it was noted in a 1998 study of navicular bone anatomy that different breeds and types of horse, as well as different types of exercise, could influence the composition of the navicular bone. So it does make some sense to suggest that changes in the navicular bone that occur as a result of stress may be part of the problem that begins what ultimately ends up as navicular syndrome. All or parts of any of the following theories may have something to do with the development of the problem.

Increased Bone Activity Theory

In 1982 in Denmark, a theory was developed which proposed that horses with navicular syndrome had bone that was more active than normal bone. This increased bone activity was theorized to be a result of increased pressure on the navicular bone. It was theorized that this pressure came from the deep digital flexor tendon where it travels over the top of the bone. (In fact, the area where the navicular bone is in contact with the deep flexor tendon is the area where most of the observed abnormalities in a diseased navicular bone occur.) According to this theory, anything that causes an increased stress on the back of the foot, such as poor foot conformation, for example, could start a horse down the road to navicular syndrome.

Interestingly, this theory of navicular syndrome also suggests that the condition is reversible if it is caught quickly. That is, if the stresses on the navicular bone can be recognized and corrected early enough, it should be possible for the bone to go back to its pre-stressed normal state. Only after secondary changes in and around the navicular bone occur (as a result of long-term deterioration of the bone) would a horse with navicular syndrome be considered incurable.

Navicular Bursitis Theory

The navicular bursitis theory, which was proposed over thirty years ago, states that the navicular bursa is the culprit. As you remember, the navicular bursa is the fluid-filled sac that lies between the deep flexor tendon and the navicular bone. It cushions the deep flexor tendon as it turns around the bone. Anyway, if the navicular bursa were to become inflamed due to repeated concussion and stress, a process of inflammation could begin that might even extend into the navicular bone and surrounding structures.

Bursitis (inflammation of a bursa) is a condition that exists in many different species: for example, in the human shoulder. Recent studies have suggested that the navicular bursa may, in fact, become inflamed in some horses. Local anti-inflammatory injections into the navicular bursa have been tried as a form of therapy (more on that in later chapters). However, navicular bursitis certainly does not seem to be a major contributor to the development of the navicular syndrome in the horses that have been studied so far.

Vibrational Theory
In the vibrational theory, proposed in 1969, the deep flexor tendon physically breaks down the navicular bone. That is, due to poor conformation (or some other contributing factor), microvibrations of the deep flexor tendon cause friction between the two surfaces (like friction generated by rubbing your hands together). Over time, this friction grinds away at the surface of the navicular bone, causing erosion of the bone and deterioration of the surface of the tendon where it touches the bone. It's an interesting idea but one that really hasn't received any serious study.

DEGENERATIVE THEORY
The degenerative theory is supported by research out of Norway. It says that navicular syndrome is a process similar to what occurs in the breakdown of joints (degenerative joint disease). In fact, the changes that are seen in the diseased bone of horses with navicular syndrome do look something like the changes that are seen in bone that comes from diseased joints. Of course, nobody knows why joints break down and become arthritic either, so while the theory is very interesting, it's not particularly helpful in understanding what is actually happening in navicular syndrome. Still, some forms of therapy are directed at treating navicular syndrome as an arthritis-like condition, with some reported success.

UNIFIED THEORY

In 1989, veterinary surgeons at the University of California at Davis proposed a theory for the development of navicular syndrome that incorporated elements of all of the above theories. Key elements of their theory include:

1. The underlying disease process is one of degeneration and deterioration of the bone, similar to that seen in arthritis of the horse's pastern (ringbone) or hock (bone spavin).

2. Abnormal mechanical forces on the foot and navicular bone cause the changes. Importantly, from a therapeutic standpoint, these forces may be altered—more on that later.

3. These mechanical forces cause the navicular bone to begin to change. Some horses may successfully make changes to their navicular bones to adapt to the stress, and never show any signs of lameness. Some horses may show occasional lameness until the bone changes its structure to accommodate the stress. However, the navicular bones of other horses may ultimately not be able to cope with the stress. These are the horses that will eventually have chronic changes in the navicular bone and become permanently lame. (Unfortunately, however, at this time there is no way to tell any of these horses apart.) But the thing to remember is that at some point in the disease process, the clinical features of all these horses may be identical—and some can get better.

4. As chronic changes occur in the structure of the navicular bone, the system of blood drainage from the bone may be adversely affected. Blood drainage may become sluggish. This poor drainage of blood causes an increased pressure inside the navicular bone. The increase in bone pressure causes the pain demonstrated by the horse.

This theory does seem to tie together a lot of the scientific knowledge that has been gained about navicular syndrome over the years. It suggests that some horses can recover from the condition if their disease process is recognized in time and the mechanical stresses on the foot are somehow altered or allowed to subside. It explains why drugs that affect the horse's circulation may be useful in treatment of the condition. Unfortunately, it also suggests that after permanent changes in the navicular bone have occurred, it may never be possible to return the horse to normal function.

Whatever theory you subscribe to, interesting new research in the field of palaeopathology (the study of disease of ancient animals) suggests that navicular syndrome is a problem that has affected horses for a long time. Researchers at the Idaho Museum of Natural History analysed fossilized navicular bones from several species of ancient horses of various sizes and found evidence that navicular syndrome has afflicted horses for millions of years. *Equus simplicidens,* the first of the one-toed horses, lived between 3.5 million and 3 million years ago. It weighed about 425 kilograms, or roughly 1,000 pounds. About 6 per cent of the 48 navicular bones that have been studied so far have lesions that could be linked to navicular syndrome. Navicular bones of the heftier, 519 kilograms *Equus occidentalis* that have been recovered from the La Brea tar pits in Los Angeles show a higher rate of equine navicular syndrome, about 21 per cent. Because lighter species of horses appear to have suffered less often from navicular syndrome than heavier ones did, researchers' findings suggest that weight also plays a role in development of the disease, which would support the mechanical theories of navicular syndrome. The presence of navicular syndrome in the bones of fossil horses that freely roamed North America millions of years ago shows that modern breeding practices and hard work can't be the only factors responsible for it.

Perhaps now you have some understanding of the complex nature of the theories of development of navicular syndrome. As you can see, navicular syndrome isn't a cut-and-dried problem. But you should be able to start seeing where therapy for horses with navicular syndrome will be directed. Treatment will be made in efforts to change the mechanical forces on the foot, to control pain and inflammation, to affect the circulation to the foot, and to control the deterioration of the bone. (All the information on how veterinary surgeons and farriers try to do this is contained in the chapters that follow.) But first, you'll want to know the steps that veterinary surgeons take to make a diagnosis of navicular syndrome. Read on!

Diagnosis of Navicular Syndrome

When a horse limps, he is said to be lame. Navicular syndrome is a cause of lameness—usually front leg lameness—in the horse. A horse that is affected with true navicular syndrome is always lame. Although this seems rather obvious, it's also very important. People overlook this simple fact. It will save you a lot of grief if you remember two simple things about navicular syndrome:

1. A horse that shows no signs of clinical lameness, that is, a horse that is not limping or shows no signs of abnormal movement, cannot be said or determined to be suffering from navicular syndrome under any circumstances.

2. You cannot successfully predict whether any individual horse is going to develop navicular syndrome using any method of diagnosis. So, for example, insofar as predicting whether your horse is going to develop navicular-related problems, conformation analysis is as useful as is reading tea leaves.

That being said, there are some important factors that have been associated with the development of navicular syndrome in individual horses. Certain diagnostic tests are used to help make a diagnosis of the development of the condition. Most, if not all, of these tests need to be used in order to properly establish a diagnosis of navicular syndrome. However, *no single test can be used to diagnose navicular syndrome in the horse.*

The proper diagnosis of navicular syndrome is not easy. For example, you can't do it just looking at a horse's foot. Nor can it be diagnosed merely by observing the way a particular horse travels (even if the horse is lame). Thus, the statement, 'Gosh, your horse is lame. I wonder if he has a touch of navicular?' is merely rash and irresponsible and mostly will cause you to lose sleep. Such a statement merely reflects ignorance on the part of the person saying it (so, don't you say it). Proper diagnosis requires careful, detailed evaluation of the horse and his lameness history.

In fact, it can often be quite difficult to distinguish between navicular syndrome and other causes of foot soreness in the horse, in particular soreness that comes from the back part of the horse's foot (the heel). Although it's relatively easy for a veterinary surgeon to localize the source of a horse's lameness to his foot, it may be a real diagnostic challenge to further pinpoint the source of the lameness to a specific structure within the foot. For example, veterinary science is currently unable to generally distinguish between a problem that might affect one of the ligaments of the navicular bone and a problem involving the bone itself (although advances in diagnostic imaging will probably make it easier to make such distinctions in the future). Or, it may not be possible to distinguish between a horse with pain coming from the digital cushion and pain coming from the deep flexor tendon in the foot.

How you choose to make a diagnosis all goes back to your definition of navicular syndrome. If you are a veterinary surgeon and you choose to lump any causes of foot or heel soreness together as a part of the navicular syndrome, then you are going to make that diagnosis in a lot of horses. If, on the other hand, you are more restrictive in your diagnosis and you limit the use of the term 'navicular syndrome' to only those problems in which it can truly be demonstrated that there has been degeneration of the navicular bone, you'll probably use that diagnosis much less often and with a lot more reluctance. Either way, it's not an easy process.

FACTORS THAT MAY PREDISPOSE A HORSE TO NAVICULAR SYNDROME

Age

Most people seem to think that navicular syndrome is a disease that affects old horses, those more than fifteen years of age. In fact, navicular syndrome is a disease of horses in the prime of their athletic life, usually from seven to fourteen years old. Horses that are less than three years old or more than fifteen years old appear to be three to five times less likely to develop navicular syndrome.

Sex

There appears to be no association with the development of navicular syndrome and the sex of the horse.

Breed

It does seem that certain breeds of horses are more frequently affected with navicular syndrome than are others. Thoroughbreds, Quarter Horses, and warmbloods seem to have a higher frequency of navicular syndrome than do other breeds. No one knows why this is so. However, navicular syndrome is also most commonly seen in athletic horses. Horses of the aforementioned breeds are those most commonly used for strenuous athletic competitions such as jumping, barrel racing, and eventing. Events such as these cause considerable stress on the horse's limbs. Therefore, it's possible that what, on the surface, appears to be a breed predisposition for the development of navicular syndrome may only reflect the activity for which the horse is used.

Genetics

There is starting to be some evidence that the shape and condition of the navicular bone (as graded on X-rays) may have something to do with a horse's parents. That's not the same thing as predicting that an individual horse is going to have navicular syndrome, but there does seem to be a connection with the shape and condition of the bone on the development of the clinical problem. But it's not a cut and dried thing; just because one horse has navicular syndrome doesn't mean that all of his offspring will. There is research going on in Holland that is attempting to document the effect of genetics.

Since the mid-1980s, one of the criteria used to approve Dutch Warmblood stallions has been a grading scale that takes into account all of the many X-ray changes that can be seen in navicular bones. In addition, a numbering system has been developed to describe the shape of the top edge of the navicular bone as seen on X-rays. Dutch horses have been followed for fifteen years to see what effect the selection process has had on the heritability of the grade given to the bone. However, there hasn't been enough time yet to see what effect the selection process has had on the heritability of bone shape.

The preliminary results are interesting. The percentage of horses with navicular bones that grade the poorest have decreased from 20 to 30 per cent down to 5 to 10 per cent in the past fifteen years. And work published in 2001 suggests that the shape of a horse's navicular bone may also be influenced by genetics (although the shape of the navicular bone has not been directly associated with the development of navicular syndrome). This information may ultimately be very important in selecting horses for breeding, although it may be less relevant to adult horses that are being considered for purchase (see Chapter 9).

Hoof Abnormalities

It's commonly thought that if a horse's foot isn't normal, he will be more likely to develop navicular syndrome. A normal foot should be of the proper length, angle, and balance for that individual horse—even for an individual leg of that horse.

Many types of abnormal feet have been described in the horse. What all these hoof factors have in common is that, at least theoretically, they may concentrate abnormal stresses on or around the heels, and by association, the horse's navicular bone. The mechanical theories of the development of navicular syndrome suggest that abnormal stresses on the horse's foot may have something to do with causing the problem in the horse. Even if it doesn't cause navicular syndrome, an abnormal hoof is certainly not a desirable thing in any horse and it can lead to chronic hoof soreness.

Proper hoof care is extremely important in any horse. It is especially so in the horse affected with navicular syndrome. There is a great deal of information about dealing with these hoof problems and caring for the foot of the horse with navicular syndrome in Chapter 6.

Conformation Abnormalities

Another thing that has been suggested as predisposing a horse to navicular syndrome is the horse's conformation. Conformation is the study of how the horse 'should' be put together in relation to how he 'is' put together. Of course, in reality, conformation is not something that you can do anything about but it's fun for some people to talk about.

Anyway, in addition to the previously mentioned foot abnormalities, many people consider a horse with upright (in relation to the ground) pasterns as being predisposed to navicular syndrome. Theoretically, an upright pastern does not bend and absorb stress as well as a more 'normal' pastern. The stress has to go somewhere, however, and the navicular bone supposedly gets more than its share of stress in these horses. Similarly, some people blame small feet for predisposing a horse to navicular syndrome. As convincing as they may sound, there aren't any studies to support these ideas, however.

NAVICULAR SYNDROME: MAKING THE DIAGNOSIS

Lameness History
The first rule bears repeating: if your horse has navicular syndrome, he must be lame. If he's not lame, he doesn't have navicular syndrome. Period.

But assuming that your horse is lame, navicular syndrome is usually an insidious thing. It often sort of sneaks up on the horse. Horses with navicular syndrome do not generally become acutely and suddenly lame. It's much more common for people to notice one of a number of little things in their horse that have become a bit worse over time.

Perhaps you have noticed that the horse with navicular syndrome has been traveling a bit 'short' on his front legs. That is, he doesn't seem to want to reach out and land on his heels in a normal fashion. Maybe a particular gait seems choppy and uncomfortable to ride. This makes sense since the navicular bone is in the heel area of the foot, and if the horse can shorten his stride he presumably won't have to land so hard on his heels. Maybe a shorter stride doesn't hurt so much. You may have even noticed that this reduction in the length of the stride has become worse over time.

(Curiously, when many people see a horse short-striding, they immediately think of a problem in the horse's shoulder. Although a sore shoulder muscle will cause a horse to short-stride because he doesn't want to stretch that area forward, shoulder problems in the horse are actually pretty uncommon. Most lameness problems in the horse originate from the front foot. If you want to venture a guess as to why a horse is lame—even so as to annoy your friends—you're more likely to be right if you guess that the problem is in the foot.)

Perhaps you've noticed that the horse's lameness has been intermittent. That is, he seems a bit lame on some days but just fine on others. This happens; horses with navicular syndrome can have good days and bad days. However, usually, if a horse has navicular syndrome, over time the lameness will progress and eventually become a constant problem for the horse.

Perhaps the horse's lameness gets worse with exercise (although this would be expected with most conditions that cause lameness) and gets much better with rest, for no obvious reason. You don't see any swelling or pain when you manipulate the leg. This is typical with navicular syndrome. Usually, with navicular syndrome, there are no obvious signs as to why the horse might be lame.

Perhaps you've observed that the horse's lameness is worse when it is turning in a circle. When a horse makes a tight circle, more of his weight is forced over the leg that lies on the inside of the circle. If a horse has a sore foot, as occurs with navicular syndrome, the increase in weight caused by the horse turning may cause it to show characteristic signs of lameness, such as flinching or bobbing his head when the affected leg hits the ground. Most horses that are affected with navicular syndrome seem to have the problem with both front feet. Therefore, it's not at all uncommon to see the horse limping on whichever front leg is on the inside of a tight circle. In fact, a circle may be the only place where lameness is evident. When the horse travels in a straight line, you may not even notice that he is limping. If both feet hurt, the poor lame horse may not even know which leg to limp on! (Think of yourself walking barefoot across a hot concrete driveway. Which foot hurts the most? Can your friends tell by looking while you're hopping along in agony?)

Perhaps the lameness gets worse when the horse is worked on hard or rough ground. Softer ground provides more cushion to the horse's foot. Harder ground would presumably make travelling on a foot that is sore as a result of navicular syndrome more uncomfortable.

All of these symptoms could be present, but so too could a very few. None of them are sure signs of navicular syndrome, either. To get a true diagnosis, you have to keep looking deeper.

Hoof Testers

A hoof tester is a deceptively simple device and something that no equine veterinary surgeon can be without. It simply squeezes the horse's hoof. If the horse jumps or tries to pull his leg away when pressure is applied to the hoof with the hoof tester, it may indicate that the horse's foot is sore in the area that was squeezed. (There is a bit of an art to this, however. Some horses will jump when just about any pressure is applied to their foot.)

A horse with navicular syndrome may react to pressure placed in certain directions with the hoof tester. Typically, horses with navicular syndrome will react to hoof tester pressure in one or all of three ways:

1. Pressure placed from the central groove (the central sulcus) of the frog to the toe.

2. Pressure placed from one of the grooves on the side of the frog (the collateral sulci of the frog) to the hoof wall on the opposite side of the groove.

3. Pressure placed across the back of the heels.

If a horse reacts to hoof tester pressure in one or more of these areas, the reaction should be consistent, repeatable, and uniform before you start considering that the response is significant and that the horse may have a problem in the area. In addition, all of the other areas of the horse's foot should be checked to make sure that they aren't painful or reactive. After all, hoof testers are hardly precise instruments; the response to the hoof tester that you observed in the heels could actually be originating from some other spot. Of course, you also want to make sure that the horse isn't just reacting to *any* sort of pressure on his foot.

Unfortunately, not all horses that have navicular syndrome react to hoof tester pressure. Even if a horse doesn't respond to hoof tester pressure, he can still have navicular syndrome. Remember, no single test can be used to make a diagnosis of this difficult condition.

Hyperextension Test

The hyperextension test is one of several types of stress tests that can be performed in the diagnosis of navicular syndrome. In this test, the horse's foot is placed on one end of a board. The other side of the board is then lifted up in the air gradually. As the board is lifted, it levers the horse's toe up off the ground.

This test should theoretically stretch out the structures on the back of the leg as the toe is lifted up off the ground. As the structures stretch, the tension in the deep flexor tendon and the suspensory ligament of the navicular bone should increase. If these areas are sore, increasing the tension should make the problem worse. The horse may demonstrate a positive response to this test by jumping off the board or by having a more obvious limp when he is trotted off. (Of course, since they aren't always the most cooperative beasts, some horses are going to jump off the board when it is elevated just because they don't like it.) Although a positive response to this test is interesting, a negative response does not rule out a diagnosis of navicular syndrome.

Frog Pressure Test

In the frog pressure test, a piece of wood, a stick, or even a hoof knife is placed under the back two-thirds of the frog of the horse's foot. The opposite leg is then held up in the air for a minute or so, forcing the horse to stand on the chunk of wood.

Standing on an object in this manner should put pressure more or less directly over the structures that lie above it, which would include the navicular bone, navicular bursa, and deep flexor tendon. If, after the opposite leg is released, the lameness in the leg that was on the object increases when the horse is trotted off, it suggests that there is some deep foot soreness. Again, like the hyperextension test, a negative response to this test does not rule out the presence of navicular syndrome and a positive test isn't conclusive.

Flexion Test

A flexion test is commonly performed to assist a lameness diagnosis of many conditions of the horse's legs. In the front leg, a flexion test is performed by holding the fetlock joint up in the air with some amount of pressure for sixty seconds or so (the amount tends to vary according to who is doing the test). Immediately after the leg is released, the horse is trotted off in a straight line. Sometimes lameness, if it existed, is made worse by this test.

The flexion test makes some horses with navicular syndrome

quite lame. This is probably because the test causes some sort of compression on the structures in the back part of the horse's pastern and foot. In navicular syndrome, some or all of these structures may be sore. Compressing may make them hurt more.

However, remember that when you flex the horse's fetlock joint, you not only bend that one joint, you also bend all the other joints of the lower limb. In addition, you compress all the tendons and ligaments that run down the back of the horse's leg. You may also adversely affect the flow of blood to the horse's leg when you hold it up in flexion. The test varies depending on such things as the age of the horse, the length of time that the leg is held in flexion, the day that you do the test, and the sex of the examiner (males tend to flex harder than females). It should therefore be rather obvious that the flexion test is not a precise test for the diagnosis of navicular syndrome—in fact, it's not a precise test for much of anything. Sometimes horses that are clinically normal and have no signs of any disease will limp after a flexion test! Still, a positive response to a forelimb flexion test can give you one more bit of information when you are trying to determine whether or not a horse has navicular syndrome.

ANAESTHETIC 'BLOCKS'
When a lame horse is evaluated, one of the most common methods used by veterinary surgeons to determine the source of the lameness involves the use of local anaesthetic agents. When a horse limps, it's because he hurts somewhere. If you can remove the source of the pain, even temporarily, the horse will immediately stop limping. Thus, the use of local anaesthetic 'blocks' that temporarily deaden areas of the horse's leg are extremely useful in helping to determine the area from which the soreness that is making your horse limp originates.

That's the good news. The bad news is that there is no nerve block that can specifically tell you that a horse has navicular syndrome. The whole process of pinpointing the source of a horse's lameness on the navicular bone would be made much easier if veterinary surgeons could be sure that when they placed local anaesthetic in a certain spot in or around the foot, they'd know that they had made just one or two things numb. However, the precise path of the nerves that actually supply the navicular bone and its various associated structures is something that has only recently been worked out. Unfortunately, insofar as coming up with a diagnosis goes, those nerves supply a number of structures in the foot. So, if you 'block' one spot, you remove the sensation from a whole group of things.

In trying to make the diagnosis of navicular syndrome, three different nerve blocks may be employed. These blocks anaesthetize many of the same areas; there's a lot of overlap. Still, each block may give the veterinary surgeon a slightly different bit of information—or at least a slightly different perspective. (Prior to reading on about nerve blocks, it may be useful to review the information about the nerve supply to the navicular bone in Chapter 1.)

It may also be useful to use more than one block. Unfortunately, because of the overlap, and because blocks may make the affected area numb for a few hours, you may have to wait for one anaesthetic block to wear off before you can do another one. This means that if your veterinary surgeon has a busy schedule, the horse that is being evaluated may have to be seen over several visits, so that each block can wear off before starting on the next one. Like most everything else about the navicular syndrome, interpreting the anaesthetic blocks is complicated.

Predictably, given the complexity of the condition, no one block is diagnostic for the navicular syndrome. It's really quite a mess. (In fact, in reading the explanations of the nerve blocks that follow, it may help to have a pencil and paper on hand so that you can try to help keep the effects of the various blocks straight!)

Heel (Palmar Digital Nerve) Block

It's relatively easy to put a small amount of anaesthetic over each of the nerves that runs down the back of the horse's pastern. This, and the fact that lameness associated with the front foot is the most common lameness of the horse, means that the 'PD' (palmar digital) nerve block is undoubtedly the most frequently performed nerve block in the horse. A horse suffering from navicular syndrome should improve dramatically from his lameness after this block is performed. And you can see a lot of things that you didn't know were there when you start blocking nerves. For example, since most horses with navicular syndrome have the condition in both front feet it's not at all uncommon for the lameness to 'switch' legs after the heels of one leg are made numb with anaesthetic. Since, after the block, the horse no longer feels pain in the one leg that hurts, it may begin to limp on his other leg (the one that is now more sore). In fact, the lameness exam may be the first time you even noticed that your horse was sore in both legs!

If you take only one thing from this book, this next sentence might be it. Almost any horse with pain in his foot, from whatever the cause, should improve with a palmar digital nerve block. *A horse cannot be said to have navicular syndrome based solely on the response to this block.* This block will remove the sensation from all of the structures in the horse's heel, as well as the bottom of his sole. A PD block numbs the majority of the horse's foot. It does not only affect the navicular bone.

Coffin (Distal Interphalangeal) Joint Block
When anaesthetic is placed into the joint of the horse's foot (the coffin joint), it makes the structures in direct contact with the joint, as well as the joint itself, numb. Thus, the suspensory ligaments of the navicular bone and the impar ligaments, as well as the nerve fibres that are carried in these ligaments (that run directly to the navicular bone) are likely to be anaesthetized by this block. Other structures in the horse's heel—including the navicular bursa, the deep digital flexor tendon, and even pain coming from the sole of the foot—can be affected as well. This may be a particular problem if you wait for 10 or 15 minutes, because, with time, the anaesthetic will continue to spread and can affect a wider and wider area. But, in general, a coffin joint block is thought to be one way to block pain coming directly from the navicular bone and/or its supporting ligaments, as well as from the coffin joint itself. Remember—and this is important—the coffin joint block cannot distinguish between navicular bone pain and pain coming from the coffin joint itself (some horses do have foot pain as a result of inflammation of the coffin joint).

After observing the results of a block of the coffin joint, a PD block would be a logical next step in helping to reach a lameness diagnosis. By using the blocks in combination you could tentatively conclude:

39

1. If the horse is better in the first few minutes after the coffin joint block but doesn't improve with a heel block, the problem is most likely to be in the coffin joint itself.

2. If the horse is better after the coffin joint block and also improves with the heel block, the problem is more likely to be deep in the foot and may involve the navicular bone or its supporting structures.

3. If the horse isn't any better after the coffin joint block and improves after a heel block, the problem is in the foot but it may not involve the navicular bone (although it could involve some of the other structures associated with the navicular bone such as the navicular bursa and deep digital flexor tendon; please read on about the navicular bursa block).

4. If the horse doesn't get better after any of the blocks, the problem is somewhere else!

Navicular Bursa Block

It is possible to place anaesthetic directly into the navicular bursa that lies between the deep flexor tendon and the navicular bone. If done properly, it appears that this block may provide some additional useful information in the diagnosis of navicular syndrome.

Honestly, though, this is not a block that is without potential problems. Since the navicular bursa is deep within the foot, the injection involves a bit of technical skill, plus some horses don't like it very much. It's very hard to know that you are actually in the navicular bursa with your needle, even when the needle is viewed directly with a fluoroscope! (A fluoroscope is an X-ray camera that lets you look inside the foot while you are sticking a needle in it.) In addition, complications, such as severe and sometimes permanent lameness, have been reported as a result of this block. Thus, some veterinary surgeons are reluctant to use it.

If the block is performed properly, it numbs the navicular bursa and the surfaces of the navicular bone and the deep digital flexor tendon (these structures make up the sides of the navicular bursa). This block can also cause a loss of feeling in the navicular bone itself if the anaesthetic is absorbed into the bone (say, for example, if the bone is thin due to deterioration caused by the disease process). And, as with the other blocks, it can also remove sensation from the sole of the horse's foot.

If it is done properly, the navicular bursa block may provide some additional specific information that cannot be obtained by using one of the other diagnostic nerve blocks. For example, horses have been seen that respond positively to a PD block and do not respond to a coffin joint block. When the navicular bursa of these horses is blocked, the horses move sound. This uncommon combination of results suggests a problem involving deterioration of the deep digital flexor tendon deep in the foot.

Radiographs

Radiographs (X-rays) are probably the most commonly used diagnostic technique for the evaluation of navicular syndrome in the horse. Portable X-ray machines are easy to use and commonly employed in lameness and prepurchase evaluations. But, oh, are radiographs of the navicular bone a source of controversy in the veterinary community!

It's really pretty easy to take X-rays of the navicular bone. Usually two views of the bone are taken during a routine exam. The first view, the 60-degree dorsopalmar shot, is taken with the horse standing on the X-ray plate (Figures 4a and 4b). The angle of the X-ray beam in this technique is approximately 60 degrees to the plate. In this shot, the navicular bone has to be viewed through the short pastern bone (second phalanx).

The second view, the 'skyline' shot, is also taken with the horse on the X-ray plate but it's taken from the back of the leg, with the X-ray beam being directed down the leg and between the heels. After exposing the X-ray film in this fashion, the radiographs are then developed and evaluated for 'changes' from normal. (See Figures 5a and 5b.)

The interpretation of X-rays is a bit of an art. It requires a lot of time, training, and experience. It's not easy to do. Although they are probably good people in their own right, your horse trainer, farrier, or best friend are not the people who should be looking at your horse's X-rays. That's the job of your veterinary surgeon.

Everyone seems to be able to agree pretty well on what an

41

Figure 4a. The 60-degree dorsopalmar (D-P) radiograph is taken in the manner shown here.

Figure 4b. The resulting radiograph of a normal navicular bone is shown as well.

unchanged navicular bone looks like on an X-ray. However, differences of opinion arise as to what constitutes an abnormal navicular bone radiograph. Traditionally, veterinary surgeons are trained to look for changes in the navicular bone such as little holes (some peo-

Figure 5a. The 'skyline' radiograph of the navicular bone is taken as shown here.

Figure 5b. This projection results in a very different view of the navicular bone (as illustrated).

ple call them lollipops), sharp looking bone spurs from the edges of the navicular bone, loss of bone density, hardened edges of bone (called sclerosis), and so on. Indeed, some horses that suffer from navicular syndrome do have such changes. The problem is, at least

Figure 6. A 60-degree D-P radiograph of the navicular bone, showing changes along the lower border of the bone. Changes such as these may be completely normal for a horse. Horses with problems in the navicular bone area may also have similar changes. However, some people would wrongly consider changes such as these a definite indication of a problem in the navicular bone area whether the horse is lame or not.

insofar as interpreting radiographs goes, so do some normal horses (Figure 6).

It's been well demonstrated that a variety of radiographic changes can exist in normal horses. Many of these 'changes' are the normal little pits and depressions along the navicular bone where the lining of the coffin joint moulds into the bone (these are called synovial invaginations by veterinary surgeons; see Chapter 1). A 1992 study of 583 horses in Germany documented numerous changes in the navicular bones of horses that showed no signs of lameness. The Dutch have found that about 15 percent of sound Dutch stallions have navicular bones that grade poorly on their 0–4 scale. Many of these changes would be almost automatically identified as abnormal by most veterinary surgeons. Studies done in England have also confirmed that there is a wide variation in the X-ray appearance of the navicular bone in clinically normal horses.

A study done in the United States in the mid-1980s is really disturbing if you'd like to hang your hat on the significance of X-rays of the navicular bone. In this study, 35 horses that had been diagnosed as being lame from navicular syndrome and fifteen normal horses were X-rayed. Of the lame horses, 70 per cent had changes in their X-rays. Unfortunately (from a diagnostic standpoint), so did 60 per cent of the normal horses! Furthermore, the veterinary surgeons who participated in the study were not able to distinguish between horses that were lame and normal horses based solely upon their X-rays.

What is apparent is that navicular syndrome is not a condition that can be diagnosed just by using X-rays. Certainly, in a horse that has all the clinical signs of navicular syndrome, X-rays can be used to help confirm the diagnosis. But some clinically normal horses have bad X-rays. Conversely, some horses that have navicular syndrome have no X-ray changes at all. So although X-rays are an important part of the diagnostic process for navicular syndrome, they must be interpreted with care and caution. X-rays alone can never be used to make a diagnosis of navicular syndrome. It should also be rather obvious, given the wide variety of changes that can be seen in the normal horse, that X-rays can never be used to tell if a horse is going to develop navicular syndrome at some point in the future (see Chapter 9).

Diagnostic Ultrasound

Ultrasound beams are sound waves that are sent into tissue. They 'echo' back from the tissue and can give an indication of what's going on inside. Ultrasound has found wide acceptance as a diagnostic technique in such areas as evaluation of tendons and ligaments, or of the equine reproductive tract, to name just a couple.

Unfortunately, ultrasound appears to be of limited value in the diagnosis of navicular syndrome, mostly because the foot is not an easy structure to ultrasound and one can't ultrasound all of the relevant structures. Still, researchers at the University of Minnesota have been able to ultrasound directly over the fleshy part of the horse's frog and see what's going on in parts of the deep flexor tendon and impar ligament in some horses. Time will tell if this technique gains wider acceptance.

Scintigraphy

Compared to such things as the lameness exam, or even X-rays, nuclear scintigraphy is a relatively new diagnostic technique for the examination of lame horses. Although the technique is readily available in most areas where there are a lot of horses, the equipment involved is quite expensive. Additionally, since scintigraphy uses radioactive material, there's a lot a government regulation involved in using the equipment. Thus, most of the scintigraphy units are found in large facilities such as referral hospitals and universities.

When a horse is evaluated by scintigraphy, it is given an injection of a radioactive material in the jugular vein. This material rapidly circulates throughout the horse's body. The horse's legs are then scanned with a camera that measures the amount of radiation in various areas. If there's a high amount of radioactivity in a certain spot, it suggests that area could be the source of the horse's problem.

Scintigraphy relies on the presence of the process of inflammation in helping to determine an area of soreness. When an area of the horse becomes inflamed, blood vessels in the area begin to leak fluid between the cells that make up the vessels themselves. (Incidentally, the leaking of fluid is also one of the reasons why inflamed areas tend to get swollen.) In a 'leaky' area of the horse's body, the radioactive material that is shot into the horse will be found in a higher concentration than in the surrounding areas. Thus, if an area of the horse shows a high level of radioactivity, that area is generally considered to be inflamed. You then work out that the inflamed area is the source of the horse's problem.

That's the good news. The bad news is that scintigraphy is not a particularly precise diagnostic technique. That is, although you use scintigraphy to help localize the general area of the horse in which a problem occurs, it won't tell you exactly what or even precisely where the problem is. Scintigraphy does not allow you to directly 'image' an inflamed area in the same manner that X-rays do. You can't use the technique to see the structures inside the horse's body. And there are problems with falsely positive and falsely negative results. Still, it's a useful diagnostic technique for the evaluation of lame horses. Unfortunately, it's not one that is guaranteed to give you an answer to your horse's lameness problem if that problem is suspected to be navicular syndrome.

Computed Tomography (CT) and
Magnetic Resonance Imaging (MRI)

Fortunately, medicine progresses and with the advances in medicine come advances in imaging techniques used to look inside diseased patients. In the case of navicular syndrome, techniques that are well established in the human field, such as CT scanning and MRI are likely to become more widely available for horses. Studies on cadaver limbs using CT and MRI have shown changes in the navicular bones, as well as the associated tendons and ligaments, which are not evident on conventional X-rays. As these devices come into greater use, it's likely that earlier and more accurate diagnoses will be made.

Response to Therapy

It should be frustratingly obvious that there's no easy way to make a diagnosis of navicular syndrome in a horse. After all your diagnostic efforts in a horse with characteristic lameness and all the typical clinical signs, it still might not be possible to say with any authority exactly what condition your horse has. Therefore, some experts suggest that a diagnosis of navicular syndrome should not be made until a horse fails to respond to any type of therapy for at least three months. Three months should be enough time for most conditions to show at least some improvement with treatment. Unfortunately, most horses with deterioration of the navicular bone don't ever get better.

Making the diagnosis of navicular syndrome in a horse is rarely easy or clear. Unfortunately, many people seem to think that it is. For example, when noticing that a horse is bit lame, some people will wonder, 'Gosh, I wonder if it has touch of navicular?' as if that were the most common cause of lameness in the horse (which is absolutely false). That's sort of like wondering if your friend, who's feeling a little under the weather, might have a 'touch of cancer'.

Even if proper diagnostic procedures are followed, sometimes the diagnosis of navicular syndrome still can be elusive. For example, a horse can be lame, have soreness to hoof testers, go sound after a PD anaesthetic block, have some changes on the X-rays, and still not have navicular syndrome. To further complicate matters, in the author's experience, all of the obvious signs of navicular syndrome

47

discussed above are rarely present in an individual horse. To tell the truth, from a diagnostic standpoint, navicular syndrome is a real pain.

Lameness involving the horse's foot—in particular, the heel—is quite common: probably the most common of all causes of lameness in the horse. Lameness involving the navicular bone is much less so. The current state of diagnostics in veterinary medicine sometimes makes it hard to separate many foot-related problems from lameness specifically associated with the navicular bone and its associated structures. However, given the poor prognosis for recovery from 'true' navicular syndrome (and the good prognosis for such things as heel soreness or foot bruising getting better), it behoves you and whoever is looking at your horse to approach the diagnostic process carefully and thoughtfully so that you don't make a big mistake. You don't want to unwittingly condemn a horse that, with a little time and treatment, just might get better.

Medical Treatment of Navicular Syndrome

Whatever the method that you use to make it, once a diagnosis of navicular syndrome has been made, you are undoubtedly going to want to try to treat your horse and make things better. You can probably guess that this is rarely an easy condition to treat, particularly if serious changes have gone on in and around the navicular bone. And, as you might expect with a condition that's as complicated and difficult to diagnose as navicular syndrome, there's no sure-fire cure. Still, medical treatment strategies are available to help control the pain of the condition as well as to try to get to one of the possible root causes of the problem. Any or all of them can be tried; none of them may work very well.

NONSTEROIDAL ANTI-INFLAMMATORY DRUGS

Nonsteroidal anti-inflammatory drugs (NSAIDs, for brevity's sake) are among the drugs most commonly used to treat navicular syndrome. Drugs of this class include phenylbutazone ('bute'), flunixin meglumine (Banamine), naproxen and aspirin, among others.

NSAIDs have two primary effects on the horse. The most obviously useful effect is the relief of pain and inflammation. Navicular syndrome causes the horse a big pain in the foot; by giving a drug that relieves pain, he may be able to use his foot in a more normal fashion. NSAIDs do not 'cure' the problem of navicular syndrome. They do, however, help to cover up the pain, and may allow a horse to be ridden more comfortably.

A second, possibly beneficial, result of these drugs is their effect on the horse's circulation. NSAIDs inhibit the formation of blood clots. This is a result of their effect on a type of blood cell called a 'platelet'. Platelets are the cells responsible for starting the blood-clotting process. (This anti-clotting effect of NSAIDs is why people who have had heart attacks are sometimes advised to take an aspirin a day. It helps prevent blood clots in the heart.) If you buy into the idea that navicular syndrome is related to problems in the horse's circulation, then giving a drug with some anticoagulant activity makes some sense. There's never been a study done to investigate whether or not the anticoagulant effects of NSAIDs are actually useful in the treatment of navicular syndrome, however.

All these drugs work in a similar fashion along similar chemical pathways, although there are differences in the ways the individual drugs work. There are certainly significant differences between the costs of the various drugs. Some horses do seem to respond better to one drug than another, so it's probably worth it to try another one if the first one that is prescribed doesn't seem to help your horse.

NSAIDs have gained an unjustified bad reputation in the horse community as being loaded with adverse side effects. Horse owners seem to be especially concerned about side effects on the horse's stomach (gastric ulcers) and kidneys (kidney failure). While it is true that these side effects have been seen in horses given NSAIDs, bad effects seem to be rare when recommended doses of the drugs are given. No drug is completely safe 100 per cent of the time. However, if you follow the recommended dosage of NSAIDs, it is extremely unlikely that you will ever see a problem in your horse, even if he is maintained on the drugs for years.

STEROIDS (CORTICOSTEROIDS)

The other potent anti-inflammatory compounds given to horses are called steroids. Actually, steroids are a whole group of compounds that have a variety of effects on the horse. Corticosteroids are one group of these chemical compounds. The particular effect of corticosteroids that is useful for treatment of navicular syndrome is their ability to strongly inhibit and suppress inflammation. By directly reducing inflammation, they also help indirectly to relieve pain associated with various conditions.

Corticosteroids may be given to a horse orally, or by direct injection into an inflamed area. Local injections are the most common method of administration of this type of drug to horses suffering from navicular syndrome. However, corticosteroids do not cure a disease by relieving inflammation. The relief obtained from steroid injections is often only temporary unless the underlying problem can be corrected.

In the treatment of navicular syndrome, two areas of the horse may occasionally be injected (in no particular order):

1. Navicular bursa injections. If there is inflammation of the navicular bursa, it may occasionally be relieved by direct injection of steroids into the bursa. This is a rather tricky procedure, however. It's actually quite difficult to place a needle between the horse's heels and into the horse's navicular bursa (although the procedure for doing so has been described in books and magazines). Direct viewing of the foot with a fluoroscope during the injection process has shown how hard it really is to do correctly. It's impossible to be 100 per cent certain that you are actually in the navicular bursa if you don't attempt to look inside the foot while you are doing the injection. Even if you do get a good navicular bursa injection, studies have shown that the beneficial effects are generally temporary.

2. Coffin joint injections. If there is pain and inflammation associated with the coffin joint or the structures associated with it (see Chapter 1), direct injection of corticosteroids into the joint may help to provide some relief to the horse. Unlike the navicular bursa injection, this injection is not at all difficult (for someone with training). Frequently, coffin joint injections of corticosteroids are combined with hyaluronic acid (another anti-inflammatory compound that is a component of normal joint fluid), in an effort to help increase the anti-inflammatory effect. Some veterinary surgeons seem to feel that injecting a horse that responds to anaesthesia of the coffin joint is always 'worth a shot'.

ISOXSUPRINE HYDROCHLORIDE

Isoxsuprine is a drug that causes dilation of the small blood vessels found in the peripheral circulation in people. These small blood vessels exist in the extremities (hands and feet) and in the brain. Small peripheral blood vessels usually carry blood that flows at very low pressure. Since the pressure driving the blood flow is so low, it's likely it can be easily stopped or slowed down by various medical conditions. In people, isoxsuprine is used to try to help dilate these small blood vessels to help relieve the effects of blood insufficiency in the brain and other tissues. Interestingly, however, the drug is considered to be only 'possibly effective' for use in people by the US Food and Drug Administration. That is, the FDA isn't sure if or how well the drug works at doing what it is supposed to do.

In the horse, isoxsuprine was first investigated for the treatment of navicular syndrome around 1980. Its use was considered because of the theories that navicular syndrome is caused by problems with blood circulation to the navicular bone. By using isoxsuprine, it was hoped that any circulation problems could be relieved by dilating the small blood vessels that are found there. By dilating the blood vessels, the circulation could be theoretically 'improved' and the problem would thus take care of itself.

Indeed, two studies showed that many horses with navicular syndrome do benefit from administration of isoxsuprine. These experimental data were supported by the clinical experiences of veterinary surgeons in the field as well. Consequently, isoxsuprine became one of the most commonly prescribed drugs for treatment of navicular syndrome in use. Still, it is curious that, after all of this time, no one really seems to know how the drug works. Perhaps if the flow of blood to the navicular bone is 'improved', the horse will get better due to a healthier environment being created for the bone. Alternatively, if the flow of blood away from the bone is 'improved' with isoxsuprine, perhaps the pressure that builds up in the navicular bone as a result of sluggish blood flow is somehow relieved. Amazingly enough, either way, no one has demonstrated that the circulation to the feet is actually affected by isoxsuprine.

And it gets even more confusing. A published report in 1998 indicated that orally administered isoxsuprine has no measurable pharmacological effect at the usual dose rate (1.2 mg/kg twice a day)! The authors of the report concluded that isoxsuprine is almost completely and immediately metabolized when it's given to horses orally and that orally administered isoxsuprine is not likely to reach effective blood levels in the horse. It has also been shown that isoxsuprine doesn't affect the blood flow to the feet—at least in healthy horses—anyway. Given the difficulty in making an accurate diagnosis, it does make one wonder if many of the horses that 'responded' to isoxsuprine simply got better, either on their own, because they were misdiagnosed in the first place, or because of other things that were done for them.

If you do try the drug for your horse, it's important to remember that the response to isoxsuprine is not dose dependent. That is, if the prescribed dose of isoxsuprine doesn't work, giving the horse more won't make any difference. The author has seen horses that have been given up to five times the recommended dose in hopes that there would be some 'extra' effect for a 'really bad' case of navicular syndrome. This just doesn't make any medical sense at all. Fortunately, the drug is very safe, so even if the recommended dose of the drug is exceeded, there are unlikely to be any side effects. (The author has seen one horse that had an apparent allergic reaction to the drug. Allergic reactions can happen with any drug, however.)

POLYSULPHATED GLYCOSAMINOGLYCAN (ADEQUAN)

If you believe that navicular syndrome is caused by deterioration or degeneration of the navicular bone (a condition much like arthritis of a joint), then it would make some sense to try a drug that is used in the treatment of arthritis. Polysulphated glycosaminoglycan (PSGAG) is a substance that is chemically similar to substances that occur in normal joint cartilage. These substances are called mucopolysaccharides. PSGAG appears to interfere with the function of enzymes that are released during joint inflammation. There may also be some effect from the drug in regard to protecting the deterioration of the joint cartilage, which occurs with arthritis. (The actual extent of that effect is being almost continuously evaluated. The jury is still out on the actual benefits of the drug.)

Anyway, if the cause of navicular syndrome has something to do with an arthritis-like deterioration of the navicular bone, then the use of PSGAG compounds to treat it makes sense. In 1993, a study was presented evaluating the use of intramuscular injections of

Adequan (a brand of PSGAG) for the treatment of navicular syndrome. (The drug is given by injection into the muscle. It is absorbed from the muscle into the bloodstream. It then travels in the circulation to the joints.) Fifteen horses were in the study, of which seven actually received the drug (the study was done 'double-blind' so that the results weren't biased). All of the horses had been lame for less than twelve months.

The investigators in this study concluded that administration of PSGAG did improve the lameness signs in the seven horses that received it (frankly, that's not a whole lot of horses). The drug was given according to the manufacturer's recommendations (one shot in the muscle every four days for a total of seven doses).

The only real drawback to this method of treatment of navicular syndrome is the expense—Adequan isn't cheap. Of course, no treatment, including this one, works for every single case of anything (that's the way things go in medicine). Still, the use of intramuscular PSGAG injections for the treatment of a horse with navicular syndrome is something you can try when other treatments don't seem to help.

There are glycosaminoglycans sold in feed stores that are intended for oral use in the horse: chondroitin sulphate and glucosamine. No one knows how well (or if) they work in the treatment of arthritis, much less for the treatment of navicular syndrome.

ANTICOAGULANTS

If you buy into the idea that navicular syndrome is caused by problems with blood circulation to the foot, another form of treatment that might make sense is the use of anticoagulants. In people who have had a heart attack or a stroke caused by blood clots, anticoagulants may be used to help prevent the formation of clots in the future. The idea behind using this sort of drug therapy in horses with navicular syndrome is identical.

The anticoagulant drug that has been most extensively evaluated for treating horses with navicular syndrome is warfarin (yes, it's rat poison). The effectiveness of treatment has been reported at anywhere from 40 to 80 per cent. It's easy to give and it's cheap.

Unfortunately, there are many disadvantages to warfarin treatment. Since the drug stops blood from clotting, you have to monitor the horse carefully to make sure that he's not getting too much. You have to take blood tests continually to make sure you haven't had too much of an effect on the blood's ability to clot. (You don't want your horse with navicular syndrome being treated with warfarin to bleed to death from a cut.) Also, bleeding in a number of sites such as the chest cavity or abdomen, joints, ovaries or the sheath of male horses (to name just a few; bleeding can be seen almost anywhere) has been seen in warfarin-treated horses. Finally, warfarin interacts with many drugs that are used to treat horses with other conditions, such as phenylbutazone, antihistamines, and corticosteroids. These disadvantages have kept warfarin therapy from being widely used in the treatment of navicular syndrome.

FUTURE DRUG STRATEGIES
Other drugs that affect the blood supply to the horse's foot may also someday be used in the treatment of navicular syndrome. Mentrenperone helps stop blood vessels from spasm and contraction; its effects are supposed to be similar to the effects of isoxsuprine. Pentoxiphylline is a drug that allows red blood cells to become more flexible and helps reduce blood clotting, but its use in horses with navicular syndrome hasn't been reported. Since nothing else seems to work all of the time, these probably will be tried in the future.

ACUPUNCTURE
Acupuncture has been resurrected from medical history rather recently and promoted as something that could be of some benefit in treating horses with just about any condition, including navicular syndrome. There's certainly no good evidence to support such a contention. Suffice it to say that the claims made for acupuncture far exceed any evidence of effectiveness. Under no circumstances— as with other purported treatments—is acupuncture a cure for the condition.

MAGNETIC THERAPY
There's been a big rush to apply magnets to just about any part of a horse that can be exposed to a magnet. Among other things, magnets are supposed to increase or improve the circulation to injured

areas of the horse. Supposedly, better circulation would allow for improved healing.

In fact, no such effect has ever been demonstrated in the horse (or any other species, for that matter), and a couple of studies have tried. Improvements or increases in circulation have not been shown in the horse. Nor has improved healing been demonstrated. The weak magnetic fields in these pads are unlikely to penetrate down to the navicular bone anyway. However, purveyors of magnetic devices or pads are doing a booming business in supplying something to people in search of a quick and easy solution to a complex and difficult problem. Although there's no demonstrable benefit to the horse from applied magnetic devices for the treatment of navicular disease, they're not likely to hurt anything except your wallet.

EXTRACORPOREAL SHOCK WAVE THERAPY (ESWT)

High intensity sound waves have been used to help break up things like gallstones and kidney stones for a number of years. The sound waves—the technique is called lithotripsy—encounter the stones and blast them into little bits. When sound waves work, it's good news because it saves the patient the time, expense and trauma of surgery.

In the mid-1980s, European investigators got the idea that the technique might be useful in treating human orthopaedic injuries. So people in Europe started getting their limbs 'shocked' for such conditions as calcifying tendonitis (where calcium deposits get laid down in tendons) or chronic heel pain. There have been a number of reports that have suggested that the treatment has had some success for these conditions. Just how the device is supposed to work is still a bit of a mystery. Suggestions have been made that it stimulates bone formation, increases circulation, and/or simply causes a temporary loss of sensation to the treated area.

Subsequently, and recently, devices intended for use in horses have started to flood the market. Among the numerous proposed applications is for the treatment of navicular syndrome. Unfortunately, so far, there haven't been any published reports of the results of the application of ESWT to horses with confirmed navicular syndrome (there are some glowing testimonials, but you can find those for just about anything). It does seem a bit hard to understand how or why the therapy might help horses with navicular syndrome. Perhaps if there is some numbing effect from the therapy, its apparent success could simply be attributed to that (of course, if the treated horses never had navicular syndrome in the first place...). The bottom line is that after fifteen or so years of using ESWT in human medicine—despite encouraging results in some indications—the lack of coherent therapy schemes and poorly designed clinical studies have seriously hindered the drawing of reasonable conclusions about its effectiveness. Studies in veterinary medicine are in their infancy.

LASERS

In the 1960s, eastern European doctors proposed that low-intensity laser light had remarkable therapeutic effects. This focused light, in intensities that are, by definition, too low to cause heating effects in tissue, was said to possess remarkable healing properties. The initial reports sparked a flood of interest in the therapy and good scientific studies were initiated. Unfortunately, good studies have generally failed to show a relevant clinical effect in humans or animals.

As far as treating horses with navicular syndrome, the use of low-intensity lasers, though advertised, seems silly. Light is absorbed, reflected, or scattered relatively quickly as it hits tissue and there's no reason at all to suppose that any amount of light gets to a structure as deep in the foot as the navicular bone. There's certainly no good evidence—and no good reason—to believe that lasers have any relevant clinical effect for treating navicular syndrome.

GALLIUM NITRATE

A particularly creative theory as to the cause of navicular syndrome proposes that high aluminium levels in feed are the source of the problem. The feed is supposedly contaminated by aluminium leached from rock by acid rain, which causes loss of bone mineral from the navicular bone and, as a result, navicular syndrome. The proposed treatment for the 'problem' is administration of gallium nitrate, which is supposed to enhance mineralization of the navicular bone and counteract the bad effects of the aluminium.

Extraordinary claims—such as above—generally require extraordinary evidence to support them before they will find wide acceptance. Suffice it to say that insofar as gallium nitrate is concerned, that evidence has not yet been forthcoming. Don't hold your breath.

REST

Time supposedly heals all wounds. Fortunately, in many cases this is true. For the treatment of lameness ascribed to navicular syndrome, time may bring about a cure in some horses as well.

If you subscribe to the theory that navicular syndrome is caused by some sort of change in the navicular bone in response to stress, some time off to allow the horse to go through those changes and get over the stress makes a lot of sense. In addition, if you are trying to do something in regard to the horse's foot in an effort to alter the stress on it, it may take time, possibly as long as six months, for that something to have an effect.

Then you have the horses that have been diagnosed with navicular syndrome but really don't have it. Some of those horses will eventually return to soundness if they are just rested long enough. Sadly, you can't predict in advance which ones they will be. The necessary amount of time for healing in these cases can be considerable. If, for example, a horse has hurt a ligament in his foot, it may take up to a year or more for that horse to return to soundness. The bottom line is if your horse has been diagnosed with navicular syndrome and it really doesn't have it (a regrettable possibility that can occur easily enough) things are probably going to get better!

EXERCISE

Yes, this treatment is just the opposite of rest. However, you can make an argument that exercise may be beneficial in some horses with navicular syndrome. Exercise has been shown to increase the blood flow to the foot. Exercise also helps to increase the effect of any shoeing treatment. (For example, if you are trying to get the horse's foot to expand with a 'corrective' shoe, making him walk on the shoe should help the shoe do its job.) Some horses with navicular syndrome may benefit from exercise, up to thirty minutes a day, after proper shoeing (see Chapter 6). However, some horses with sore feet just get more sore if they are worked, so you have to give exercise a try and see what happens.

Unfortunately, in some horses with navicular syndrome no amount of therapy is going to return them to soundness. Not only does no one treatment for navicular syndrome work on every horse, some horses won't respond to any treatment at all. If, as a result of disease, structural changes have taken place in and around the navicular bone, the horse it not going to get better. If, for example, scar tissue has formed between the navicular bone and the overriding deep flexor tendon, no amount of time is going to take away that scar tissue. These poor horses will have a permanent lameness problem to deal with. How to care for these horses becomes part of the philosophy of dealing with a horse that has navicular syndrome (see Chapter 8).

CHAPTER

6

Horseshoeing Strategies for the Treatment of Navicular Syndrome

Whatever else you might have to say about navicular syndrome, there's no arguing that the problem affects the horse's foot. And for better or worse, man can manipulate no part of the horse as much as the foot. So, inevitably, the foot gets a lot of attention when it comes to the treatment of navicular syndrome. By trimming the foot and applying various shoes, pads, and other devices, people make efforts to right the wrongs that they perceive in their horses.

Good foot care and corrective horseshoeing can help many horses with navicular syndrome get better. Unfortunately, there's no single way that's guaranteed to help every horse. Furthermore, some horses can't be helped with any form of shoeing or trimming. Still, it's good to be aware of the many suggested forms of horseshoeing care available for the horse with navicular syndrome so that you can try as many things as possible.

THE NORMAL FOOT

In order to work out if your horse has any problems in his feet, you should consider what the horse's foot is supposed to look like and how it works. Then, if your horse doesn't fit the 'normal' picture, you can take some strides to get him there.

Hoof Angle

If the bottom of the foot is on level ground, the front part of the hoof wall forms an angle with the ground (and the bottom of the foot). For most horses, the normal angle of the front foot is between 50 and 55 degrees. (Some people will tell you that the angle should be lower than this, something of the order of 45 degrees. That's just not right, according to all of the studies that have been done.)

Individual horses can vary within this normal range. There's no correct angle for every horse (not every person wears the same size shoe, either). Horses can even have a different angle for each foot and still be normal.

The correct angle for a horse is said by some people to be the same as the angle from the withers to the point of the shoulder. While that may be true, it's not the easiest measurement to make, particularly on, say, a fat horse with no withers. An easier, more commonly used way to see if the horse has the proper hoof angle is to look to see if a line drawn along the front of the hoof wall is parallel with a line running through the middle of the pastern to the ground. This angle is most easily seen when the horse is viewed from the side with the horse standing on the foot in question. This line is called the hoof/pastern axis (Figure 7).

Once the hoof is trimmed so that there is a straight line from the pastern to the ground, you can pick up the hoof and measure the angle. Gauges are available to do just that. Your farrier should have

Figure 7. The angle of the foot (measured along the front of the hoof wall) and the hoof-pastern axis (measured down the middle of the pastern, from the fetlock joint to the ground) ideally should be identical.

61

one. If not, get one yourself. Keep records. Even though it takes a few minutes, you want to do all you can to keep problems from occurring in your horse.

Foot Length

The length of the foot is pretty important, as well. There has to be enough foot to cover and protect the sensitive structures underneath the hoof from impact with the ground. If a horse's foot is too short, he's going to feel the same way that you would if you ran around barefoot on the pavement all day. A short foot can get sore and bruised very quickly. Conversely, a foot that is too long may make the horse stumble or trip. The length of the foot is measured from the hair at the coronary band (from where the hoof grows) to the ground at the toe, at the front of the foot. It's been done that way since the days of Alexander the Great (really!), so it's a time-honoured way of measurement.

Like foot angle, the proper foot length differs for each individual horse. Still, some general guidelines have been developed for foot length:

1. For smaller horses—between 800 and 900 pounds—the toe length should probably never be shorter than three inches.

2. For medium-sized horses—between 950 and 1,050 pounds—the toe length should probably never be shorter than $3\frac{1}{4}$ inches.

3. For larger horses—those over 1,150 pounds—the toe length should probably never be shorter than $3\frac{1}{2}$ inches.

Make sure you don't overlook the length of the foot when your horse is being evaluated for lameness. The length is an easy measurement to make. If the length of the foot isn't appropriate for your horse, you may end up with problems that could be confused with navicular syndrome.

Balance

The balance of the horse's foot describes a relationship between one side of the foot and the other. It's commonly felt that it's ideal, though not always possible, that one side of the foot be the same length as the other side. The top of the foot (at the coronary band) should look parallel to the ground when viewed from the front, and the heels should be the same length when viewed from the side. Finally, when a properly balanced foot is picked up, half of the foot should be on either side of the frog (Figure 8). Once a foot is balanced, the foot should ideally land flat when it hits the ground and not on one side or the other.

Balancing a foot is indeed a noble goal. The true importance of minor imbalances in the hoof is a subject for discussion, however. Studies have shown that by changing the side-to-side balance of the foot, you actually do very little to alter how the stress is applied to it. No matter what the side-to-side balance, the inside heel on the front leg receives the most stress during a stride. Furthermore, as the foot grows, the balance that you started with can change. However,

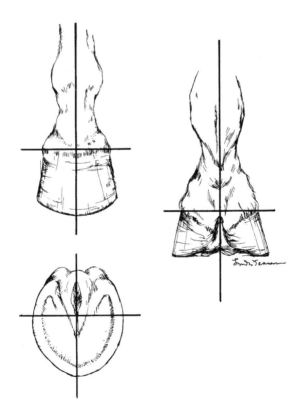

Figure 8. When ideally trimmed, a foot should be symmetrical and balanced when seen from the front, the back and the bottom.

even though its actual importance to the horse can be difficult to assess, a properly balanced foot is still a good thing to shoot for.

Heels

As mentioned before, the heels of the horse's foot take quite a pounding. Accordingly, there are some people who feel that the more heel a horse has, the more protection will be given the foot and the better off he will be. To some extent, this is probably true. Horses with low or no heels have been shown to have a variety of ailments associated not only with the foot but with the whole lower leg.

However, more is not necessarily better. While a horse should have an adequate amount of heel, it's important to keep the idea of balance and proper angle in mind, too. A horse can have too high a heel; that's not any better than one that is too low. Keeping a horse's heels long is not necessarily a good idea and certainly no way to prevent a horse from developing navicular syndrome.

SHOEING THE HORSE
WITH NAVICULAR SYNDROME

Correcting Pre-existing Abnormalities

It goes without saying that proper shoeing and trimming and good hoof care will go a long way towards helping to keep your horse sound. Unfortunately, most horses don't have a perfect, 'normal' foot. Of course, the feet they come with are the only ones they have, so you just have to make the best of them.

Prior to applying any sort of artificial protective device or shoe to the foot, it's important to trim the foot to make it as close to 'normal' as possible. You'll be surprised how many horses do better when their foot has simply been trimmed and shod correctly. Still, it's generally thought that certain hoof abnormalities are associated with the development of navicular syndrome in a horse. Some of the specific abnormalities include:

1. **A broken hoof/pastern axis.** The hoof/pastern axis is an imaginary line that can be drawn through the horse's lower leg when the leg is viewed from the side (as discussed earlier). A line drawn through the centre of the hoof and pastern intersects with the flat line of the ground and can be seen to

Figure 9. This horse has a broken back hoof/pastern axis.

make an angle with the ground. This line should be parallel to the normal angle of the hoof. (See Figure 9.)

If the horse's foot is at an improper angle, the normal straight line that should be seen in a properly trimmed foot doesn't exist. Instead, the line bends or breaks at the coronary band of the horse's hoof. If the horse's heels are too high, the line (the axis) will be broken forward. Conversely, if the heels are too low, the axis will be broken back.

Neither of the above abnormal situations is desirable for the horse. Proper trimming, by raising or lowering either the toe or the heel, helps ensure that the horse has an unbroken hoof/pastern axis. You want to try to make sure that the foot has the proper angle for that particular limb.

2. **Underslung (some people use the term 'underrun') heels.** Research has shown that when a horse strides, he normally lands with the majority of his weight on the heels. A horse with low or underslung heels has little hoof tissue under the back part of the foot to absorb his weight when he moves. If

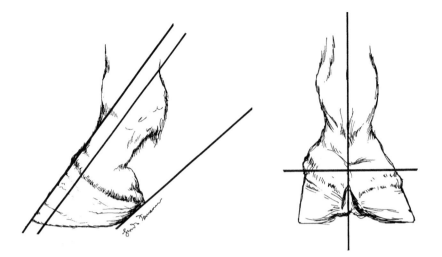

Figure 10. This horse has a mildly underslung heel.

Figure 11. This horse has sheared heels.

the horse's heel is abnormally low, the sensitive and important structures of the back part of his foot may take an increased pounding. This almost certainly predisposes a horse to developing sore heels. It may also be associated with the development of navicular syndrome. (See Figure 10.)

It's difficult to correct a horse that has underslung heels. Obviously, you can't make a horse grow more heel by cutting on that part of the foot. However, you can help restore some of the normal angle of the foot by working on the horse's toe. Over time, generally many months, it may be possible to help a horse grow some heel by trimming and shoeing, but you're unlikely ever to turn a really bad foot into a good one. However, until such time as the horse does grow some heel, often some sort of artificial device, such as a pad, is used to help protect, cushion and sometimes even raise, the heels.

3. **Sheared heels.** The heels of a horse's hoof are said to be sheared when one of the two heels on the hoof is noticeably higher than the other. In addition, the hoof wall on the higher heel is usually more vertical than normal. The hoof wall on the

more normal heel also tends to flare out. (This is most easily seen when the hoof is viewed from behind.) Contrary to popular belief, conformation appears to have something to do with sheared heels, it's probably not a result of bad shoeing. Sheared heels have been associated with heel soreness in some horses, and according to some people, it may be associated with the development of navicular syndrome. (See Figure 11.)

Correcting sheared heels can be quite difficult and, if a horse is moving normally, it may not be all that important. In any case, corrections are not something that can be accomplished in a single trimming. Most farriers try to take pressure off the heel that is too high ('floating' the heel) in an effort to get it to drop lower to the ground. Meanwhile, the rest of the foot is balanced and supported with some sort of shoe, such as a bar shoe (discussed later in this chapter).

4. **Contracted heels.** Contracted heels are heels that are pinched too close together. In fact, the whole foot in a horse with contracted heels often tends to be narrow, almost like the foot of a deer. Although it's a somewhat subjective assessment, if the heels are too close together, it indicates that the foot may not be expanding and contracting properly with the normal movement of the horse. If the foot doesn't work properly, it would seem less likely to be able to relieve the stress applied on it. Thus, contracted heels appear to be a cause of chronic heel soreness and, possibly, may lead to the development of navicular syndrome.

Correcting contracted heels is a time-consuming process. In fact, it can be quite difficult to do if the horse is kept in shoes at all! By taking the horse out of shoes altogether, spreading of the foot is encouraged. Some people even go so far as to encourage the horse to stand in water or mud in an effort to soften the feet and help them spread out. (How well this sort of thing works is anyone's guess.) A variety of corrective shoeing methods are also described for the treatment of contracted heels, such as placing springs between the heels in an effort to push the walls out or the use of 'slippered' shoes (see p. 73).

Some horses are born with a foot in which the heels are contracted. Others develop the problem over time, as a result of trimming and shoeing. Horses that develop contracted heels due to trimming and shoeing seem to be easier to return to normal by good hoof management than are horses born with the problem.

5. **Small feet** (on a big horse). Small feet are not something that can readily be changed. It's theorized that a small foot on a big horse takes more stress than a bigger foot would. More stress supposedly increases the likelihood that the horse will develop navicular syndrome.

    About the only thing you can do for this 'problem' is to shoe the horse with as large a shoe as possible. (Of course, not all large, small-footed horses will develop navicular syndrome.) You also want to set the shoe wide to allow for maximum expansion of the foot. Then, cross your fingers.

6. **Improper trimming and shoeing** is a man-made addition to the stresses that are normally placed on a horse's foot. A full discussion of horseshoeing theory is beyond the scope of this book. However, some general rules for proper shoeing and trimming of the horse's foot are:

    a.   The trimmed foot should be level from side to side.

    b.   The trimmed foot should be balanced from front to back, from side to side, and on the bottom.

    c.   The trimmed foot should be of an appropriate length and at the proper angle.

    d.   The sole should be cupped as much as practical. That is, the sole should be trimmed out so that when weight is placed on the foot, it can expand.

    To demonstrate this effect, put your hand on a counter or tabletop. Make sure that you place it in a relaxed fashion, leaving a small cup in your palm. You can hit the back of your hand surprisingly hard (within reason) with your other hand without causing any pain. This is because the 'cup' of your hand flattens and expands and helps to spread out the shock applied to it. The horse's hoof is supposed to work in the same fashion.

e. The heels should be properly supported by extending the heels of the shoes as wide and as far behind the foot as is practical.

f. Nails placed in the foot should not be placed behind the widest part of the foot. This should help to make sure that the foot, especially the heels, can expand.

Pads

The idea behind putting a pad on a horse's foot is disarmingly simple. If the foot hurts, why not put some sort of cushion between it and the shoe to help absorb the shock and protect the foot? If you can soften the blow on the horse's foot, hopefully the horse will move better. In fact, many times pads do help horses with sore feet, even horses whose foot soreness can be traced to navicular syndrome.

Pads are made from any one of a number of materials, including rubber, plastic, leather, and numerous synthetic compounds. They come in an endless array of designs, many of them accompanied by various claims as to how their particular style or material makes them especially effective. It's a bit bewildering to try to deal with all the pads and all the claims out there. Clearly, there's no single best pad, or everyone would be using it. Like so many things about navicular syndrome, your best way to approach the question of which pad to use is to try a bunch of them.

Not only does the type of material used to make a pad vary, but the shape of the pad can vary as well. For example, some pads are designed to alter the pressure on various parts of the foot. This effect is especially obvious with pads that have an insert built in to apply pressure to the frog. Applying frog pressure theoretically will increase the amount of weight that the frog has to carry. This can be of benefit to horses with sore heels. In the author's experience, however, frog pressure doesn't seem to help (and occasionally hurts) horses with navicular syndrome.

Wedge pads are one of the most common types of pads used for the treatment of navicular syndrome. A wedge pad is just what it sounds like: a wedge of material that is higher on one end than the other. Two types of wedge pads are made, one that completely covers the horse's foot, and another that can be inserted just between the back part of the shoe and the horse's heels. Wedge pads are thought to have several effects:

1. By elevating the heel, it is hoped that strain (tension) on the deep flexor tendon is relieved. Raising the heel would, in theory, relax the deep flexor tendon. (It would tend to straighten out the tendon.) Hopefully, this could help decrease the pressure put on the tendon by the navicular bone as the horse bears weight on his leg.

2. By elevating the heel, some cushion may be provided to the heel area. This tends to soften the impact in the whole area.

3. By elevating the heel, breakover is improved.

Not everyone thinks that wedge pads are always a good idea, however. In some horses, it seems as if the pads actually compress and destroy the heels over time. Thus, other methods of heel elevation may be employed. These include building the heel up with acrylic hoof repair material, thickening the heel area of the shoe itself by doubling it over ('swelling' the heels of the shoe), or using a premade shoe that is already elevated.

Breakover is a term that refers to how the horse's foot leaves the ground. For a horse to get his foot off the ground, he must rotate the foot over the toe (breakover) as the leg travels forward. Theoretically, if you elevate the horse's heel, it tends to push the foot up and forward. The foot can't sink as low into the ground when its heels are elevated with some sort of a wedge as it otherwise might. This effect would tend to make the foot break over the toe more quickly, at least theoretically. For the horse with navicular syndrome, this might mean that the horse would stay on the heel for less time and the forward movement of the foot would be made a bit easier.

Investigations have shown that elevating a horse's heel does tend to increase the breakover of the foot. Unfortunately, it's not a consistent effect. Some horses don't change their breakover when their heels are elevated. Furthermore, breakover changes are not consistent with all gaits. That is, just because the breakover is faster at the walk doesn't mean that it will be faster at the trot and canter as well.

As a final consideration about elevating heels with wedges, remember that in using them, you don't necessarily just want to jack up the horse's heels. You do want to maintain some sort of balance to the foot and maintain a normal hoof/pastern axis. Therefore, some people recommend that if, for example, a wedge pad is used to treat a horse with navicular syndrome, the foot should first be trimmed to the proper angle and then lowered by 3 degrees. A 3-degree wedge pad is then applied to the foot to restore the normal angle and provide the benefits mentioned above. Frankly, although this sort of treatment does seem a bit odd (why not just keep the foot at its normal angle?), it apparently helps some horses with navicular syndrome.

Basically, like most everything else about navicular syndrome, you may have to try some sort of a pad or some method of heel elevation on your horse's foot and see if it works. If it doesn't work, try something else. Every change you make is likely to do something. However, you might not be able to predict what that something is. (Understand that you might not be able to find anything that works, either.) Nobody is going to get it right the first time, every time.

Corrective Shoes

In addition to the various pads used to treat horses with navicular syndrome, a variety of horseshoes intended to correct the problem are prescribed. The variety seems endless.

The ancient Romans initially devised horseshoes as a method of keeping horses' feet from wearing out. For this purpose, they work very well. However, in addition to this basic function of horseshoes, a seemingly infinite array of 'corrective' horseshoes has been described to treat and correct various conditions of the foot. Farriers are remarkable in their ability to shape iron. The horse's foot often benefits from a creative approach to farriery.

Horseshoes can be something of a double-edged sword, however. While it is true that they protect the foot, they also have the potential for causing harm. Being rigid objects, horseshoes tend to inhibit the natural expansion of the foot. In addition, they tend to concentrate the stress on the foot along the shoe (particularly in the nail holes). As such, they tend to make the wall of the hoof bear more of the weight of the horse than the rest of the foot; normally, all foot structures participate in weight-bearing. Therefore, it's obvious (and very important to realize) that an improperly applied horseshoe may be much worse than no shoe at all.

For the treatment of navicular syndrome, one of several types of horseshoe may be prescribed:

1. **Egg bar shoe** A bar shoe is one that places a complete ring of metal underneath the horse's foot. It's closed at the horse's heels by a metal 'bar' (as opposed to the 'normal' shape of the horseshoe that you would have over your door for good luck). An egg bar shoe is shaped much as the name would imply, with the 'bar' of metal extending well back behind the horse's heels.

   The main way to tell that an egg bar shoe is properly applied is if it can clearly be seen from the widest part of the foot extending back behind the heels. In addition, the bar of the shoe should extend back to the bulbs of the heels (the bulbs are the soft, fleshy part of the heels just below the coronary band). The point to which the bar should extend back can easily be seen when a line is drawn from the bulbs of the heels perpendicularly down to the ground. Egg bar shoes seem to be very useful for the treatment of horses that have underslung heels. (See Figure 12.)

   Unfortunately, it's been shown that egg bar shoes don't do anything to reduce the pressure on the navicular bone and they may make the horse's gait slightly less animated. It's also possible to put on an egg bar shoe that's too long. Some people feel that a too long egg bar shoe may act as a lever on the heels and crush them. In addition, if the shoe is too long, the horse can more easily pull it off. A bit of trial and error may be inevitable.

2. **Rolled toe shoe** If you look at a shod foot from the side, you can see that there is a flat layer of metal nailed on to the bottom of the foot. The thickness of the horseshoe increases the effective length of the horse's foot. This could, in theory at

Figure 12. This is a properly fitted and placed egg bar shoe.

least, help to slow down the breakover.

In an effort to help the horse with navicular syndrome break over his toe (and get off his heels), some people recommend that the toe of the corrective horseshoe be rolled. For example, the toe of the shoe can be rounded off with a grinder. A shoe with a rounded or rolled toe certainly gives the impression that the horse should be able to roll more easily over the front of it than with a normal shoe. As an alternative to rolling the toe, some horseshoes are made from 'half-round' steel; that is, in which the metal bar of the shoe is already rounded.

To increase the effect of rolling the toe, some people recommend an even more dramatic change. By taking off some of the toe with a hoof rasp and bending the toe of the horseshoe up at the slight angle, a 'rocker' toe can be made. This may help speed up breakover even more.

3. **Slippered heel shoe** In an effort to increase the expansion of the foot, sometimes the heels of the shoe can be 'slippered'. This means that the back part of the shoe is ground down at an angle, leaving the highest part of the shoe on the inside part of the foot and the lowest part of the shoe on the outside of the foot. Slippering the shoe will, it is hoped, help the foot to expand by causing it, in effect, to slip down the ramp that

Figure 13. A shoe with slippered heels, such as illustrated here, theoretically will help promote expansion of the heels.

has been created at the back of the shoe. If a pad is used on the horse's foot that can be slippered, too. (See Figure 13.)

4. **Tennessee navicular shoe** This type of colourfully named, premade aluminium shoe has reportedly helped some horses with navicular syndrome. It's a type of bar shoe. The shoe elevates the heels due to its deep metal branches, and also protects the heels with a bar of metal.

5. **Wide-web shoe** These shoes are made out of a piece of metal that is wider than the 'normal' horseshoe. It places more metal under the horse's foot, which presumably provides more protection. One advantage of the wide-web shoe is that it can easily be set so as to extend beyond the edges of the hoof wall. This is of particular advantage when you are trying to help a horse with a small foot.

Just as with pads, when you are nailing (or even gluing) shoes on to the foot of a horse with navicular syndrome, you may have to try a number of things until you find something that works (if you are lucky enough to find something that works). Plus, there are undoubtedly many other types of horseshoes advocated for the treatment of horses with navicular syndrome that haven't been mentioned here. Try them if you want to. No one knows something that is going to work every time for every horse. You will have to be patient and trust the experience and expertise of the people trying to help your horse with navicular syndrome if you intend to find the best way to shoe him.

SPECIFIC SHOE AND PAD COMBINATIONS THAT HAVE BEEN RECOMMENDED FOR THE TREATMENT OF NAVICULAR SYNDROME

The most successful approach to shoeing a horse with navicular syndrome is to take each horse individually. Each horse is going to respond differently to your treatment (that's one of the really frustrating things about treating horses). Still, you can follow two general rules.

First, you want to try to correct any abnormality of the foot that you can recognize that may be contributing to your horse's problem. This requires some time, care, and expertise on the part of your farrier and veterinary surgeon. Insist that they work together (after all, you're footing the bill).

Second, you want to try to help the normal functions of the foot. Do things to help improve weight bearing and absorb the shock and forces placed on the foot. In general, you want to help the foot expand, to support and/or cushion the heels and try to help the horse breakover his toe.

Many different ways can be tried to accomplish these things. Some specific shoe and pad combinations that can be tried to treat a horse with navicular syndrome include:

1. Trim the horse's foot normally. Apply an egg bar shoe.

2. As above, with a pad.

3. As above, with a wide-web shoe and/or pad.

4. Trim the horse's foot 3 degrees lower than his correct angle. Raise the heel back up with a 3-degree wedge pad. Apply a shoe, making sure the heels are properly supported and the nails are properly placed (as mentioned earlier in this chapter). Roll the toe of the shoe and slipper the heels.

5. Trim as above. Apply a 3-degree aluminium bar shoe. (Tennessee navicular shoe).

6. Raise the heels of the foot to above the normal angle with a pad, and roll the toe of the shoe.

7. Build up the heels with acrylic hoof repair material. Then fit the foot with a properly fitting shoe.

Unfortunately, a lot of finger-pointing goes on in the horse world when it comes to shoeing horses. Everyone seems to have an opinion about the 'proper' way to shoe your horse. They are also more than ready to share their opinion with you (whether you ask for it or not). Of course, when your horse has a serious problem such as navicular syndrome, the chorus of advice only gets louder. Unfortunately people have a tendency to start pointing fingers at the person who 'must' have caused the problem in the first place.

The best way to deal with all the various conflicting opinions that you are undoubtedly going to receive is to be proactive in caring for your horse's hoof. Get your farrier and your veterinary surgeon working together. Ask your farrier to take measurements of your horse's hoof at each trimming. (It might take a couple of extra minutes, but it's well worth it and your farrier shouldn't mind if he's interested in doing a good job.) Keep records. Be ready to try various different types of horseshoes and pads; no one knows what is going to work for any given horse. Then, when you get unsolicited and unqualified opinions from your friends and neighbours, you can smile and politely nod (maybe even rub your chin in interest), secure in the knowledge that you are doing the best you can.

Surgical Treatment of Navicular Syndrome

In some horses—those that do not respond to any sort of medical treatment or horseshoeing strategy—surgical intervention is the last step. Many veterinary surgeons are reluctant to recommend a surgical solution to navicular syndrome. That's probably for a couple of reasons. First, the decision to do surgery is something of a tacit admission that there's nothing else that can be done. Second, surgery doesn't always work.

Still, surgery is a reasonable option for some horses with navicular syndrome. Of course, once you've decided to do surgery, which surgery do you do? There are several to choose from. In the author's opinion, the ultimate decision as to which surgery to do should be based on the following three things:

1. The likelihood that the surgery will work (and the possibility of side effects).

2. The speed with which you want the horse to return to work.

3. How much the surgery costs.

NEURECTOMY

Without question, the most commonly performed surgery for treatment of navicular syndrome, at least in the United States, is cutting the palmar digital nerves that run to the horse's heels. This is called a neurectomy. It's nothing new—neurectomies have been performed in horses for over 200 years. It's a surgery that's not particularly difficult to do and one that can even be performed on a standing horse. Many techniques for performing the surgery have been described, including using a surgical laser to cut the nerves. The 'best' technique seems to be mostly a matter of the one that the person doing the surgery feels most comfortable with.

A neurectomy is the surgical equivalent of sweeping dirt under the rug. It does nothing to get rid of the problem in the navicular bone area. It only removes the sensation of pain from the horse. It's a quick and easy solution (generally) to the problem. It's a solution that allows many otherwise chronically lame horses to return to normal work. Many horses can return to work in just a few weeks after surgery. Unfortunately, it's a solution that's only temporary because the nerves will ultimately grow back.

Neurectomies seem to generate a lot of controversy in the horse world. Like most things, it's neither as good nor as bad a solution as most people would have you believe. There are a lot of things that people say about neurectomies that fly in the fact of reality. Before you can make a reasonable decision about whether or not to perform a neurectomy on your horse, you should know all the facts.

1. A horse will retain some feeling in his foot after a neurectomy. However, he won't be able to feel the majority of his foot, including the heels. He will feel the front part of his foot and know where the foot is and how to place the foot precisely and in a coordinated fashion after surgery. Most horses are not prone to stumbling or other signs of incoordination after a neurectomy.

2. The nerves will grow back. After you cut the nerves to the heels, they will try to grow back together (all injured tissue tries to heal itself, even nerves). This can happen as soon as six months after surgery. Even though it's been tried, so far no method of treating the cut nerve ends to stop regrowth of the nerves has been successful. (People have gone to great trouble to try to keep the nerves from growing back. For example, in 1994, a technique was tried where the cut ends were buried in a hole drilled in the pastern bone. So far, however, this technique has not received general acceptance in the surgical community.)

Still, you can reasonably hope that your horse will have some good, relatively long-term, relief after a neurectomy surgery. According to one study, approximately 57 per cent of horses will be pain-free for three years after a neurectomy.

3. There are some complications. As with any surgical procedure, bad things can happen. Complications are not common but you should be aware of them. Complications of neurectomy include:

Neuroma As was mentioned above, after a nerve is cut, it tries to heal itself. While trying to heal, the cut ends of the nerve can grow into an uncoordinated mass of live nerve tissue. This neuroma, as it is called, can be very painful for the horse.

In an effort to stop neuroma formation, some vets have recommended that horses be maintained on anti-inflammatory drugs for a period of time after surgery (there's no good evidence that this works, however). Sometimes direct injections of anti-inflammatory corticosteroid compounds can help relieve the pain of a neuroma once it forms. Still, sometimes another surgery has to be done to cut the neuroma out.

Infection As with any surgery, there's a risk of infection at the site where you make the incision in the skin. Proper surgical technique makes this complication pretty unlikely.

Infection of the Hoof Wall You have to keep a close eye on the horse's hoof after a neurectomy. (You should watch your horse's hooves carefully anyway.) Theoretically, it's possible to get an abscess going in the heel, from foot trauma, a nail, or the like. The abscess could go unrecognized, since the horse doesn't feel his heel, and he won't react to what would otherwise be a very painful problem. If you're not paying close attention, a serious infection could develop in the hoof.

Ruptured Deep Flexor Tendon This complication is quite serious but, fortunately, also quite rare. Mostly, this complication speaks to the necessity of being very careful to make sure that you have an accurate diagnosis prior to performing a neurectomy. If there's some sort of a tendon problem in the foot (as opposed to a problem with the navicular bone, for example) and you remove the feeling to the heel, the horse will begin to use his foot normally. Prior to surgery, the horse limped in an effort to keep weight off his injured leg. Normal weight bearing may be too much for an injured tendon. The strain of the horse's full weight can cause a damaged tendon to pull apart. There's not a great deal that can be done for the horse after this occurs.

Failure to Desensitize the Heels In some frustrating horses, even though there is no apparent lameness after local anaesthetic nerve blocks over the palmar digital nerves, cutting the nerves does not relieve the lameness. This may be because instead of there being a single nerve trunk going to the heel, some horses can have little nerve branches off the main nerve. If you fail to recognize and cut these branches during surgery, the procedure won't work. Of course, no horse should be considered for a neurectomy if he doesn't respond to anaesthetic placed directly over the nerves that are to be cut.

OTHER SURGERIES FOR THE TREATMENT OF NAVICULAR SYNDROME

Since the relief obtained from a neurectomy is only temporary, veterinary surgeons have looked for other methods to try to obtain some more permanent relief from the pain of navicular syndrome. Unfortunately, none of them has demonstrated any consistent effectiveness in the treatment of the condition. Even if these surgeries aren't in general use, if somebody brings them up, at least you'll know what they are.

Suspensory Ligament of the Navicular Bone Desmotomy

In England, a technique for cutting the two suspensory ligaments of the navicular bone has been described as a treatment for navicular syndrome. (In medical terms, cutting a ligament is called a desmotomy.) The idea behind this surgery is that if you cut the suspensory ligaments, tension on the navicular bone somehow may be relieved. After surgery, the horses are returned to work after about three months.

Initially, reports of the success of this surgery were quite encouraging. As many as 70 per cent of the horses that received this surgery recovered successfully, according to the initial reports. Subsequently, however, nobody else has been able to come up with the same good results. So far, suspensory ligament desmotomy has not found wide acceptance as a surgical alternative to neurectomy for the treatment of navicular syndrome.

Navicular Bursa Lavage

If you have reason to believe that the navicular bursa is a significant source of inflammation in a particular horse, then treating the bursa makes some sense. Lavage means to rinse something out. Lavage of the navicular bursa is a surgical procedure in which needles are stuck into the bursa so that it can be rinsed out. Any inflammatory by-products would be thereby washed out of the area. If this treatment is going to work, the lameness should improve immediately and one rinse should do the trick. Even though the treatment has been described, nobody has written any reports on its effectiveness, and the risks of this difficult procedure might even outweigh the potential benefits.

Inferior Check Ligament Desmotomy

The inferior check ligament is found just below the horse's knee. It is a strap of tissue that attaches the middle part of the deep flexor tendon to the bone behind the horse's knee. It thereby helps to keep the deep digital flexor tendon from stretching too far when the horse bears weight on his leg.

Surgeries to cut this ligament are commonly performed in young horses with an upright foot (called a club foot). By cutting the ligament, the deep flexor tendon is allowed to stretch and relax. This allows the leg to sink into a more normal position. Some people have suggested that adult horses with extremely upright hooves have an increased incidence of navicular syndrome. Accordingly, this surgery has been tried in a few cases in an effort to try to improve the upright conformation.

The surgery and aftercare are pretty straightforward and horses can get back to work in a couple of months. The surgery is assisted by corrective shoeing changes. Like navicular bursa lavage, there are no reports of how well or if this surgery works for the treatment of navicular syndrome.

Fasciotomy

In 1986, some German veterinary surgeons proposed that damage to the palmar digital nerves supplying the navicular area is part of the problem with navicular syndrome. They suggested that if you just relieve pressure and inflammation around the nerves, the condition would improve. Accordingly, a surgery was devised to dissect away any loose subcutaneous tissue or scar tissue from around the nerves (this is called neurolysis). The veterinary surgeons suggested that this technique worked best in horses early in the course of their disease and with few changes on their X-rays.

This is another surgery that hasn't been well studied. Even if it does work, it may be because manipulation of the nerve can cause a temporary loss of nerve function (a sort of short-term neurectomy). It's not a surgery that can really be recommended until more study is done.

As you can see, navicular syndrome is not really a condition for which there is an effective surgical solution. However, for most horses afflicted with chronic pain and lameness, a neurectomy, even with its potential complications, offers the surest bet of the quickest return to normal function, even though that return is only temporary. (Once lameness returns, the surgery can usually be done again.) As with everything else, there just aren't any good simple surgical answers to the complex problem that is navicular disease.

The Prognosis and Philosophy of Caring for a Horse with Navicular Syndrome

It's a lot easier to talk about what to do with a horse that has navicular syndrome if you don't own one. It's a lot easier to make dispassionate arguments about what you can do to and for a horse with navicular syndrome if you don't have any emotional attachments to him. Owning a horse is a responsibility. You are the custodian of another being's life. Decisions are best if they are well thought out and not made in the heat of emotion. In any regard, it helps to know what you and your horse may be in for if your horse actually has navicular syndrome. In the author's opinion, there are three things that you must always keep in mind when dealing with this complex problem.

1. **Diagnosis may be difficult.** In most cases, an accurate diagnosis of navicular syndrome can be time-consuming and difficult to achieve. Your veterinary surgeon may have to make several visits over a period of time to come up with a proper diagnosis. Most afflicted horses will not be so obvious as to have all of the diagnostic signs discussed in Chapter 4.

    If a diagnosis of navicular syndrome comes easily to someone, be suspicious. Your friends, your horse trainer, or even your farrier should not be the ones helping you make a diagnosis. Anyone who looks at a horse and suggests that he has a 'touch of navicular' is just being careless. Diagnosis should be done carefully and thoughtfully.

    Finally, realize that since diagnosis of navicular syndrome can be so difficult, some mistakes are going to be made by the people looking at your horse. Some horses are going to be improperly diagnosed. You might find that with a little time and patience, a little treatment and care, your horse may make a complete recovery from some other condition of the back part of the foot that was wrongly labelled navicular syndrome.

2. **Treatment can be frustrating and expensive.** As you have seen, there are many different strategies for treating horses with navicular syndrome. You may have to explore several different avenues before you find one that works. You may have to wait for several weeks to see if any particular treatment is going to be effective. Or you may not find one that works at all.

   The point is, if the first treatment that your veterinary surgeon mentions doesn't work, don't think that he or she is some sort of idiot. Don't assume that because the first shoe that you apply doesn't work, your farrier is incompetent. Let them try any one of a number of things. Get them working together for your horse. Unfortunately, some horses with navicular syndrome don't respond to any treatment.

3. **'To cut or not to cut?'** In some horses, surgery may be your last option, albeit an unfortunate one. However, the ultimate question may be, 'Do you want to be able to use your horse or not?'

If you are content to have a lame horse, or one that can't be ridden hard without coming up limping, then there's no need for surgery (or any other treatment, for that matter). If you don't mind having a big pet that you can't ride, don't cut on him. Go and buy another horse. If, however, you want your horse to perform at his previous level, surgical intervention, generally in the form of a neurectomy, may be the only way that you can get there, even if the effects of the operation are only temporary. The surgery is not cruel. Nevertheless, it is also not a cure. It may be the best that you can do for your horse.

CHAPTER 9

Prepurchase Examinations and the Navicular Bone

Prepurchase examinations are a part of the regular job for most veterinary surgeons who specialize in equine medicine. Understandably, people who are buying a horse want to do whatever they can to make sure that the horse they are buying will be able to do whatever task is intended for him. Nobody wants to buy a horse that has (or is going to have) problems. Consequently, they turn to horse experts to conduct a thorough examination of their prospective horse prior to purchase. The final arbiter of a horse's suitability is generally the veterinary surgeon.

In most prepurchase evaluations, the horse is given a thorough physical examination that concentrates primarily on the state of his legs. The length of time spent evaluating the horse's legs during a prepurchase examination is only natural. Horses are generally pretty healthy. They usually don't have things like heart problems or epilepsy to limit their use. However, they have a multitude of problems affecting their legs. These problems can cause a horse to be unable to do whatever it is that is asked of him. Since horses are used mostly for riding, one of the goals of a prepurchase evaluation is to try to discover if any of those problems exist in a particular horse. Among other things, veterinary surgeons look for abnormal swellings, areas of pain or surgical scars (that might indicate a previous neurectomy, for example) in an effort to get a clue as to what problems a horse might have.

Many people don't seem to be happy just knowing what problems a horse might have. They also want to speculate on what problems might lie in the future. Because navicular syndrome is such a problem for horses, they especially want to make sure that their new horse doesn't have it and isn't going to get it. These people want to be able to predict the future. Unfortunately, predicting the future is one thing that can't be done.

Here's a simple fact. *There is no way to tell if a particular horse is going to develop navicular syndrome.* If the horse doesn't have navicular syndrome when you purchase him (and even that can be hard to tell), you can't tell if he's going to get it in the future. Nevertheless, people still want to try to predict what's going to happen to the horse over time.

During prepurchase evaluations, one of the most commonly requested examinations is a radiographic (X-ray) evaluation of the navicular bone. This is done in a sincere but misguided effort to tell if the horse has, or is going to develop, navicular syndrome in the future. This can't be done. (Please review the section in Chapter 4 about navicular bone radiographs. As you remember, it's becoming apparent to most vets that navicular syndrome cannot be diagnosed in a horse just by taking X-rays of the navicular bone.)

The author presented a study at the meeting of the American Association of Equine Practitioners in 1994 that specifically looked at the significance of X-rays of the navicular bone in prepurchase evaluations. The study looked at 85 horses and followed the horses for at least one year after they were purchased. All of the horses had navicular bone radiographs taken at the time they were purchased. The navicular bones were 'graded' for the degree of the 'changes' that were seen in them. The study then tried to see if changes in the navicular bone could be used to predict which of the horses would subsequently develop lameness problems related to the navicular area.

Three of the 85 horses evaluated showed some signs of lameness associated with the heel area of the foot; only one of those three did not get better on his own. What was the bottom line? It wasn't possible to make any predictions about lameness in a horse's future based solely on the changes in navicular bone X-rays. The radiographs were not useful predictors of whether or not a horse would develop navicular syndrome.

So what do you do? Should you take radiographs of your horse's navicular bones prior to purchase? In the author's opinion, there are only two reasons to take radiographs of the navicular bone (or indeed, any area) during a prepurchase examination.

One reason for taking radiographs would be if you suspect that a particular area of the horse is a source of soreness for him. If a horse limps on a leg during the examination and your veterinary surgeon can find an area that he or she suspects to be the source of the lameness, radiographs may be a useful way of determining if there is a problem there. However, a prepurchase examination is not the same thing as a lameness examination. In a prepurchase examination, the veterinary surgeon is usually trying to determine 'if' rather than 'why' a horse is lame. By taking a few random radiographs, you might not even be examining the area of the horse that hurts! You might not be able to find out why the horse you are considering buying is lame. Most people don't want to do (or pay for) a lameness exam on someone else's horse.

The second reason for taking radiographs during a prepurchase evaluation is to have a record of how the horse looked at the time you bought him. There are a couple of reasons that you might want to do this. For example, you might want to have some sort of record of how the horse looked at the time of purchase so that you can have something to compare with if a problem develops down the line. If the horse is being purchased with the idea that it is to be resold in the future (and hopefully make the buyer some money), a set of radiographs, including radiographs of the navicular bone, can be a good selling point and a demonstration of good faith, especially if the horse has never had any problems.

Along the same line, a set of radiographs can be useful insurance in a horse that is intended for resale. Just because you know that navicular bone radiographs are meaningless in a normal horse does not mean the next person will. 'Normal' navicular bone radiographs (radiographs that don't show any 'changes') generally will not get you into any trouble if you intend to resell your horse. However, you will undoubtedly hear about it if your horse's navicular bone radiographs are somehow deemed to be less than ideal. Only you can assess how much risk you run of not being able to resell your otherwise sound horse if his navicular bone radiographs don't pass someone else's assessment of what's normal.

So how do you sum this up? Navicular bone X-rays mean nothing in a horse that's moving sound at the time he is examined. You may want a record of how the horse looked at the time that you bought it, but that's your decision. Remember, you can't tell if a horse is going to go lame by looking at his navicular bone radiographs. If you are gong to try to predict a horse's lameness future, looking at the radiographs of his navicular bone is just as good as a crystal ball, tea leaves, or any other method.

EPILOGUE

The diagnosis and treatment of navicular syndrome in the horse is not easy. It appears that there may be more than one cause of the condition. The diagnostic techniques currently available to the veterinary surgeon are relatively crude and not at all specific to the navicular bone. Because the techniques currently available for diagnosis are not adequate to make an accurate and immediate diagnosis of navicular syndrome, two huge problems occur.

First, many horses that do not have navicular syndrome are diagnosed as having it. This gives the impression that navicular syndrome is a problem that occurs in many more horses than it actually does. As a result, some horses may be condemned or discarded because of a condition they don't really have.

Second, it's difficult to prescribe an appropriate cure for a condition you can't accurately diagnose. You can't target a specific therapy at a condition if you can't describe the condition. Furthermore, you can't give an accurate prognosis if you don't know how bad things really are inside the foot.

You may have to try many therapies if your horse develops navicular syndrome. Therapies may include any or all of the treatments discussed in the preceding chapters: medicinal, shoeing, or surgical. If it ever becomes possible to match a specific therapy to a specific disease process, the success of treatment is likely to improve.

So, knowing all of that, be ready for a frustrating time if your horse does develop navicular syndrome. Consider all your options and do what you think is best, even if it ultimately means that you have to get another horse. As a practising veterinary surgeon, the author is just as frustrated with the state of diagnosis and treatment of navicular syndrome as you undoubtedly are. We can hope that future discoveries will make the whole process more satisfying.

BIBLIOGRAPHY

Balch, O.K. et al. 'Locomotor Effect of Hoof Angle and Mediolateral Balance of Horses Exercising on a High-Speed Treadmill: Preliminary Results.' *Proc. 37th AAEP* (1991): 687–705.

Bowker, R.M., K.K. Wulfen, and D.J. Grentz. 'Nonselectivity of Local Anaesthetics Injected into the Distal Interphalangeal Joint and the Navicular Bursa.' *Proc. 41st AAEP* 41 (1995): 240–2.

Bowker, R.M. et al. 'A Silver-Impregnation and Immunocytochemical Study of the Innervation of the Distal Sesamoid Bone and its Suspensory Ligaments in the Horse.' *Eq. Vet. J.* 26 (1994): 212–19.

Dik, K.J. and J. Van den Broek. 'Role of Navicular Bone Shape in the Pathogenesis of Navicular Disease: A Radiological Study.' *Eq. Vet. J.* 27 (1995): 390–3.

Dyson, S. 'Comparison of Responses to Analgesia of the Navicular Bursa and Intra-Articular Analgesia of the Distal Interphalangeal Joint in 102 Horses.' *Proc. 41st AAEP* 41 (1995): 234–9.

Flint, M.E., H.G. McDonald, and L.C. Østblom. 'Equine Navicular Syndrome: A Historical Perspective on a Modern Problem.' *Journal of Vertebrate Paleontology.* 2001; 21(Aug. 22):50A.

Gabriel, A., S. Jolly, J. Detilleux, et al. 'Morphometric Study of the Equine Navicular Bone: Variations with Breeds and Types of Horse and Influence of Exercise.' *J. Anat* 1998; 193 (Pt. 4): 535–49.

Harkins, J.D., G.D. Mundy, S. Stanley, et al. 'Absence of Detectable Pharmacological Effects After Oral Administration of Isoxsuprine.' *Eq. Vet J.* 1998; 30(4): 294–9.

Ingle-Fehr, J.E., and G.M. Baxter. 'The Effect of Oral Isoxsuprine and Pentoxifylline on Digital and Laminar Blood Flow in Healthy Horses.' *Vet. Surg.* 1999; 28:154–160.

Jackman, B.R. et al. 'Palmar Digital Neurectomy in Horses: 57 Cases (1984–1990).' *Vet. Surg.* 22 (1993): 285–8.

Kainer, R.A. 'Clinical Anatomy of the Equine Foot.' *Vet. Clin. NA Eq. Prac. 5* (1989): 1–27.

Kaser-Hotz, B., and G. Ueltschi. 'Radiographic Appearance of the Navicular Bone in Sound Horses.' *Vet. Radiol. and Ultrasound* 33 (1992): 9–17.

Keegan, K.G., D.A.Wilson, J.M. Kreeger, et al. 'Local Distribution of Mepivacaine after Distal Interphalangeal Joint Injection in Horses.' *Am J Vet Res* 1996; 57(4): 422–6.

Ostblom, L., C. Lund, and F. Melsen. 'Navicular Bone Disease: Result of Treatment Using Egg-Bar Shoeing Technique.' *Eq. Vet. J.* 16 (1894): 203.

Pool, R.R., D.M. Meagher, and S.M. Stover. 'Pathophysiology of Navicular Syndrome.' *Vet. Clin. NA Eq. Prac.* 5 (1989): 109–29.

Ramey, D.W. 'The Navicular Bone and Future Lameness: A Retrospective Study of Prepurchase Examinations in Practice.' *Proc. 40th AAEP* (1994).

Rose, R.J. et al. 'Studies on Isoxsuprine Hydrochloride for the Treatment of Navicular Disease.' *Eq. Vet. J.* 15 (1983): 238.

Steckel, R.R. 'The Role of Scintigraphy in Lameness Evaluation.' *Vet. Clin. NA Eq. Prac.* 7 (1991): 207–38.

Trotter, G.W. 'Therapy for Navicular Disease.' *Comp. Cont. Ed.* (Sept. 1991): 1462–6.

Turner, A.S., and C.M. Tucker. 'The Evaluation of Isoxsuprine Hydrochloride for the Treatment of Navicular Disease: A Double Blind Study.' *Eq. Vet. J.* 21 (1989): 338–41.

Turner, T.A. 'Diagnosis and Treatment of Navicular Syndrome in Horses.' *Vet. Clin. NA Eq. Prac.* 5 (1989): 131–44.

Turner, T.A. 'Navicular Disease.' In *Current Practice of Equine Surgery,* edited by N.A. White and J.N. Moore. Philadelphia: J.B. Lippincott, 1990.

Turner, T.A., and C. Stork. 'Hoof Abnormalities and Their Relation to Lameness.' *Proc. 34th AAEP* (1988): 293–7.

Turner, T.A. et al. 'Radiographic Changes in the Navicular Bone of Normal Horses.' *Proc. 32nd AAEP* (1987): 309–14.

Widmer, W.R., K.A. Buckwalter, J.F. Fessler, et al. 'Use of Radiography, Computed Tomography and Magnetic Resonance Imaging for Evaluation of Navicular Syndrome in the Horse.' *Vet Radiol Ultrasound* (2000); 41(2): 108–16.

Wild C., M. Khene, and S. Wanke. 'Extracorporeal Shock Wave Therapy in Orthopedics.' Assessment of an Emerging Health Technology. *Int J Technol Assess Health Care,* (2000); 16(1): 199–209.

Willeman, M.A., H.H. Savelberg, and A. Barneveld. 'The Effect of Orthopaedic Shoeing on the Force Exerted by the Deep Digital Flexor Tendon on the Navicular Bone in Horses.' *Eq. Vet. J* 31 (1999): 25–30.

Wright, I.M. 'Navicular Suspensory Desmotomy in the Treatment of Navicular Disease: Technique and Preliminary Results.' *Eq. Vet. J.* 18 (1986): 443–6.

INDEX

Page numbers in **bold** refer to illustrations